# THE CAMBRIDGE MEDICAL SERIES

### GENERAL EDITORS

## SIR CLIFFORD ALLBUTT, K.C.B., M.D., F.R.S.
### REGIUS PROFESSOR OF PHYSIC

## SIR WALTER FLETCHER, K.B.E., M.D., F.R.S.
### FELLOW OF TRINITY COLLEGE

# WAR NEUROSES

T0381901

# WAR NEUROSES

BY

## JOHN T. MacCURDY, M.D.

PSYCHIATRIC INSTITUTE, WARD'S ISLAND, NEW YORK
LECTURER ON MEDICAL PSYCHOLOGY
CORNELL UNIVERSITY MEDICAL SCHOOL
NEW YORK

WITH A PREFACE BY

## W. H. R. RIVERS, M.D. (LOND.)

FELLOW OF ST JOHN'S COLLEGE, CAMBRIDGE

CAMBRIDGE
AT THE UNIVERSITY PRESS
1918

# CAMBRIDGE
## UNIVERSITY PRESS

University Printing House, Cambridge CB2 8BS, United Kingdom

Published in the United States of America by Cambridge University Press, New York

Cambridge University Press is part of the University of Cambridge.

It furthers the University's mission by disseminating knowledge in the pursuit of education, learning and research at the highest international levels of excellence.

www.cambridge.org
Information on this title: www.cambridge.org/9781107626522

© Cambridge University Press 1918

First published 1918
First paperback edition 2013

*A catalogue record for this publication is available from the British Library*

ISBN 978-1-107-62652-2 Paperback

# PREFACE

THE account of the neuroses of war set forth in this book was written primarily for the instruction of the medical profession in America. Dr MacCurdy came to this country in 1917 to inquire into the nature of the problems which were about to confront the neurologists and psychiatrists of America through the participation of that country in the war. The experience he gained was originally recorded in the "Psychiatric Bulletin" of the New York State Hospitals in July, 1917, and the Cambridge University Press are greatly indebted to the editors of this journal for their permission to make Dr MacCurdy's work accessible to the public in another form.

The book describes the experience of one with a long record of skilful investigation of the psycho-neuroses of civil life when brought into contact in British hospitals with the special forms of neurosis which are produced by the shocks and strains of warfare. The cases on which the book is based are not startling rarities especially selected to show features of scientific interest, but are characteristic straightforward cases such as may be met with by the score in any hospital especially devoted to functional nervous disorders. The merit of the book lies, not in the nature of its material, but in the skill with which this material has been treated and the clearness with which the essential facts have been set down and utilized to illustrate the special problems presented by the neuroses of war.

The great frequency of functional nervous disorders in the present war has made a subject which was formerly a somewhat narrow speciality one with which every practitioner of medicine has been forced to become familiar. Dr MacCurdy's book should go far to enable him to make good use of this familiarity. The book, however, should not appeal to the medical profession alone. There are now many who are trusting greatly to the assistance of the laity when, after the war, the task is undertaken of putting the treatment of the neuroses and psychoses of civil life upon a new basis. Dr MacCurdy's book is so written that any intelligent layman will be able to follow its essential lessons. It should thus be most useful in following up the movement for the instruction of the laity already set on foot by the admirable work of Professor Elliot Smith and Mr T. H. Pear[1].

One of the lines upon which the book will exert a strong educative influence lies in the clearness and definiteness with which it brings out the essentially psychological character of the war neuroses. In the early days of the war the medical profession, in accordance with the materialistic outlook it had inherited from the latter part of the nineteenth century, was inclined to emphasise the physical aspect of the antecedents of a war neurosis. As the war has progressed the physical conception has given way before one which regards the shell explosion or other catastrophe of warfare as, in the vast majority of cases, merely the spark which has released long pent up forces of a psychical kind. Dr MacCurdy's book should contribute greatly to progress upon these lines. His cases not only bring out clearly the great part taken by purely mental factors in the production of the war neuroses, but they also show to how great an extent the symptoms of neurosis are determined by mental factors, even when the main agent in the production of the neurosis is concussion or fatigue.

In coming into touch with the neuroses of war Dr MacCurdy was especially struck by their simplicity as compared with those of civil practice. He rightly ascribes this to the fact that the war neuroses depend essentially on the coming into

[1] *Shell Shock*, by G. Elliot Smith and T. H. Pear, Manchester University Press.

play of the relatively simple instinct of self-preservation, while the neuroses of civil life largely hinge upon factors connected with the far more complicated set of instincts associated with sex. Dr MacCurdy agrees with other observers that sexual factors take a comparatively small place in the production of the war neuroses, but he believes that those who have shown a lack of adaptability to the stresses dependent on sex are also liable to fail in their adaptability to the stresses of warfare.

The classification of the war neuroses adopted in the book is one which is now coming into vogue in this country, in which two main varieties are recognised. In one the various mental factors tending towards neurosis produce states of anxiety, with symptoms similar to those which accompany anxiety in its milder and non-pathological forms. Dr MacCurdy speaks of this group in general as "Anxiety states," and does not use the "Anxiety neurosis" and "Anxiety hysteria" of other writers. He does so in order to include cases, of not infrequent occurrence, which, in spite of the presence of pronounced anxiety, can hardly be regarded as examples of true neurosis. The second group in the classification of the book is formed by those cases in which the mental factors find expression in manifestations resembling in some measure those produced by a wound or other physical disability. This group is entitled "Conversion Hysterias" on the ground that the morbid psychical energy to which the neurosis is primarily due has been converted into the physical symptom or symptoms.

Dr MacCurdy shows that the direction taken by the morbid psychical energy underlying the neurosis depends largely upon the nature of the desires entertained by the soldier before his breakdown. Perhaps the most original feature of his work is the view, duly supported by evidence, that those who suffer from anxiety states have wished for death during the period of strain and fatigue preceding the final collapse, while sufferers from conversion hysteria have entertained the desire for disablement, for a "Blighty" wound, or for some disabling illness. It is a striking fact that officers are especially prone to the occurrence of anxiety states, while privates are the chief victims of hysterical manifestations. Dr MacCurdy explains this fact by differences of education and responsibility which produce a different mental outlook towards the two chief means of escape from the rigours and horrors of warfare.

One of the most pleasing features of the book from the practical and humanitarian points of view is to be found in its attitude towards prognosis and treatment. Coming direct from practice with the neuroses of civil life, Dr MacCurdy was especially struck by the amenability of the war neuroses to treatment, provided this treatment is of the right kind.

In the early stages of the war the treatment used in this country was largely dictated by the physical conception of the neuroses and consisted chiefly in the prescription of massage, electricity and drugs. Where these remedies acted as means of suggestion, they did a certain amount of good in many cases, but too often they merely accentuated the disease, and even produced new manifestations, by encouraging the patient to believe in the physical character of his condition. The noxious influence of the uncritical administration of drugs is well brought out by Dr MacCurdy's observation that "in those hospitals where reliance is placed chiefly on drugs there is a constant difficulty in combating insomnia, whereas the difficulties are much less in those institutions where drugs are largely taboo."

While Dr MacCurdy holds that hypnotism and suggestion may be useful in demonstrating to the patient that lost or disturbed functions are not vitally affected, he sums up strongly against the general employment of these measures as therapeutic agents. He attaches great importance to the line of treatment, which following Captain W. Brown may well be called "autognosis," in which the patient is given insight into the processes by which his state has been produced. The patient is led to see that he has not been altogether the creature of circumstance, but that his own tendencies have not been without influence in the production of his state. Dr MacCurdy's main method is in fact that of re-education which in this country will always be associated with the names of Maghull under Colonel R. G. Rows and of Craiglockhart under Major W. H. Bryce.

W. H. R. RIVERS.

*July* 1918

# CONTENTS

# WAR NEUROSES

## CHAPTER I

### INTRODUCTION

WAR NEUROSES may be defined as those functional nervous conditions arising in soldiers, which are immediately determined by the conditions of modern warfare, and have a symptomatology whose content is directly related to war. Naturally enough, in any large body of troops, neuroses (as well as psychoses) develop as they do in times of peace, and many of these are determined by factors which are essentially those of civilian life. In these latter the symptoms are the same as those occurring in peace times, and can therefore not be called war neuroses with any clinical accuracy. This group of functional nervous diseases presents no problems that are different from those which have been studied for many years, and they will therefore receive no attention in the preliminary clinical report which follows.

The war neuroses, however, offer problems very new and of great importance both from medical and military standpoints. The term "shell shock" has been adopted officially by the British War Office as the diagnostic term to cover all neuroses arising among officers and soldiers of the armies. This term has an advantage in its picturesqueness that has helped to stimulate popular as well as professional interest, but it is a term which can be defended with difficulty from a purely medical standpoint. There are two reasons why this is so. In the first place it implies a single etiology—the physical effects of high explosive shells on those subjected to bombardment, who suffer no external physical injury—and this is far from being even the main factor in the determination of the symptoms. Secondly, the clinical types covered by this blanket diagnostic term are too various to be safely gathered under one heading. It is therefore more advisable to use the term "war neuroses," which gives the desired latitude in grouping together the different clinical pictures that occur, and focuses the attention on those influences which come directly from warfare.

In most countries, at the outbreak of the present war, a situation was in existence that was distinctly inimical to the careful study of functional nervous diseases. Neurotics, with their tendency to superficial recovery and frequent relapses, were insoluble problems to the bulk of the profession who were not especially trained in their treatment, so that they had become the *bêtes noires* of most general practitioners and of many neurologists. Being little understood, the general ignorance as to causation led to the adoption of hypotheses concerning the essential nature of these conditions, which were more strongly held than scientific accuracy would justify. This was, of course, a natural consequence of the multiplicity of physical and psychological factors that are probably always at work in the production of peace neuroses.

Neurotics, too, demand so much time of the physician in treatment that a tendency had developed to regard their symptoms as purely imaginary, somewhat spurious, or at least of less importance than obviously organic medical problems. The average medical practitioner naturally preferred to give his attention to concrete physical disabilities rather than to impalpable and subjective symptoms. When the war appeared, therefore, the medical attitude toward neuroses was one of rather narrow bigotry on the part of most of that small group interested in functional nervous diseases, and of indifference on the part of the bulk of the profession. Naturally then, there were few observers who were really competent to study the great mass of material which the war suddenly produced.

These thousands of cases presented problems which were no less important from a military than from a medical standpoint, and hypotheses as to their essential nature were put forth with as much enthusiasm and as little accuracy as the importance of the problem, on the one hand, and the lack of preparation on the part of the observers, on the other, would naturally be expected to produce. Those who had had little sympathy with the neurotic looked on these victims of war as mere malingerers and advised treatment by a firing squad—"pour encourager les autres." Those who had been previously interested in hereditary defects asserted that these new patients were practically all inferior individuals. Those who had emphasized physical factors in peace times were able to demonstrate to their satisfaction that all the cases were suffering from extreme physical fatigue, concussion from high explosive shells, or poisoning with gases from the explosives. On the other hand, there were those, who had worked with neurotics from a psychological standpoint, who took the ground that the war neuroses were essentially psychic in origin. As a result of this, a large literature has grown up which must be rather chaotic for the average reader to whom it is accessible, since few publications are to be found which give any broad survey of the clinical material, or a careful study of all possible factors. It therefore seemed advisable to make a survey of these cases, bearing constantly in mind the possibility of all the above mentioned factors coming into play, in order that their relative importance might be gauged as a basis for the further study and treatment of these conditions as they arise in the American expeditionary forces.

# CHAPTER II

## TYPICAL CASES

In order to orient the reader at the outset with the nature of these neuroses, it may be well to note cases representative of the two main types which are to be found. These are conditions of anxiety on the one hand, and of simple conversion hysteria on the other.

Case I. The following history is typical of the development and symptoms of an anxiety state. The patient was a man of 27 who had never been ill in his life. He had never shown any neurotic tendencies, having been entirely free from night terrors as a child, and had suffered from none of the fears or inhibitions so constantly met with among neurotics in peace times. He had never had any fear of high places, or thunder-storms, or crowds, or entering tunnels, and had had no sensitiveness to bloodshed. He had been a normal, mischievous boy, had played many games, and had been successful in his work, both in school and when he entered business life. The only abnormality to be found in his make-up was a certain shyness with the other sex, from which he had never entirely freed himself. It was perhaps for this reason that he was unmarried and had never thought of taking a wife. It is interesting to note that he always despised those who developed neuroses of any kind, and when he went to France had similar disrespect for those suffering from "shell shock."

He enlisted as a private in October, 1914, and adapted himself pretty well to the training, making many friends among his fellow soldiers and enjoying the work at first, although he became rather bored with the routine before his five months of training were completed. In February, 1915, he went to the firing line in France. In his first experience of shell fire he broke out with a cold sweat with fear, then became rather slow and depressed, without any energy, and felt rather sleepy. This reaction, however, was only temporary. He soon became accustomed to bombardment and the sight of wounds and death, and then began to enjoy his work, particularly the active operations. After eight months in the trenches he was invalided home with nephritis. He was convalescent for four months, and was recommended for a commission, which he received after two months training. Two months more being spent in his regimental depot, he returned to France as a lieutenant in June, 1916. Then followed four months of very heavy fighting on the Somme, during which time he developed no symptoms whatever. He was wounded very slightly once. One day he was buried three times by earth thrown up from shell explosions. The last time he was unconscious for ten minutes. He was relieved for three days after this experience, although he had no symptoms. He was very frequently knocked out for short periods by the concussion from shells. About the end of October, 1916, he was sent to the Ypres section where he was working with a pioneer battalion and had to bury many dead. This has been, since the outset of the war, the most trying part of the whole British line. Not only has bombardment been practically constant from the beginning, but to add to the other horrors of the situation it has never been possible to bury all the dead. In this disagreeable situation he began, after a month of these new duties, to dislike the work, and became mildly depressed, although he paid no particular attention to his feelings. Then some fatigue set in, and he found himself for the first time since his initial experience of shell fire with a tendency to jump nervously when the shells came. To keep himself in hand he began to drink. After a couple of weeks he found that his sleep was becoming poor. It took him a long time to get to sleep, during which time the scenes on the Somme front were constantly in his mind. He had a feeling that he had to get up to the trenches on the Somme the next day, and that he did not want to go. During this period of half-sleeping, half-waking, he suffered from "hypnagogic" hallucinations; that is, visions of the trenches, shells, and so on, accompanied by insight that they were really not there, but only imaginations. These visions produced no fear and at this time he had no nightmares. Matters grew worse. Every week he became more nervous; fear of the shells grew on him, he lost the ability to tell by the sound where each was going to land, and all of them seemed to be coming at him. In the effort to "quiet his nerves" he got to drinking quite heavily by the beginning of the present year. He struggled constantly to prevent any outward signs of his fear betraying his condition to his men. This effort increased his fatigue. The horror that he felt when first confronted with the bloodshed of battle, to which he had long since become accustomed, reappeared at this time. He became sensitive to all the sights that were forced on his eyes, would think of them when alone and not actively engaged on some duty, and would see them before him on falling off to sleep. He was so discouraged that·he began to wish he might be killed.

He was able to continue, however, until March, when on a raid one day seven men around him were killed and he was immediately afterward buried himself. After this he felt so much worse that he applied to the doctor, who told him he had some fever and gave him a "pick-me-up." He "carried on" for two days, but with extreme difficulty; then his condition became so bad that he was forced to report to his physician again, and was sent to a hospital. For two or three weeks he had had bad headaches back of his eyes, and his sleep had become very limited as he would constantly awake with a jump.

As soon as he got into the hospital he began having nightmares which were typical of the anxiety state. In them he was back on the Somme front and being shelled mercilessly. Shells would come closer and closer to him, finally one would land right on top of him and he would awake with a shriek of terror. After a long time he would go to sleep again, to be almost immediately reawakened with another of these dreams, the content being always the same and confined to fighting, in which he was invariably getting the worst of it.

He would awaken in the morning feeling weak, absolutely

played out. Any noise would be interpreted as a shell and strike him with terror. He was therefore suffering from a combination of fatigue and extreme nervousness, with the war constantly in his thoughts. At night when falling off to sleep he would have "hypnagogic" hallucinations of Germans entering the room, and with these visions, too, there was great terror.

After being a little over a week in different hospitals in France, he was transferred to London. There his condition greatly improved, his fatigue lessened, he became less sensitive to noises and his nightmares largely disappeared. He was next sent to a hospital in the country where he had every opportunity for outdoor exercise and recreation and continued to improve for two weeks. Then came the news of the death of one of his best friends in France, which depressed him considerably. Shortly after this a concert was arranged at the hospital and he tried to sing, but failed. This experience made him much worse. The old dreams began to destroy his sleep with great regularity. He became more disheartened and hypochondriacal, complained that he was in a sweat day and night, that he had lost twelve pounds and that he was never going to get well because his physicians would not give him an opiate. (As a matter of fact, at this time his sleep was fairly good.) He could not be induced to leave the hospital and would not go out of doors for a week at a time. He felt so much weaker that he was no longer able to play golf. He was in general quite convinced that he was physically and nervously a permanent wreck.

This case is typical, except for the occurrence of the relapse with depression.

CASE II. This case illustrates a simple hysterical conversion. The patient is a private of 20 years of age, who is not quite so normal as the individual whose history has just been cited. Although he had never had any neurotic symptoms, he showed a tendency to abnormality in his make-up. He was rather tender-hearted and never liked to see animals killed. Socially, he was rather self-conscious, inclined to keep to himself, and had not been a perfectly normal, mischievous boy, but was rather more virtuous than his companions. He had always been shy

with girls and had never thought of getting married. All of
these seclusive tendencies, however, were quite mild in degree.
The one physical trouble from which he ever suffered was a sore
throat a year or so before the war began. At this time he was
unable to sing or to talk loudly without hurting his throat. He
had always had a lisp.

He enlisted in May, 1916, and spent five months in training.
This proved to be distinctly advantageous, for he adapted himself well to it and was mentally more comfortable than before,
as was shown by his increasing sociability. On going to the
front, October, 1916, he found himself frightened, as is usual, by
the first shell fire he encountered, and horror-struck by the
sight of wounds and death, but soon became free from fear and
quite accustomed to the horrors around him. After five months
of fighting, he was sent to Armentières in March, 1917, and had
to fight for three days without sleep. He became tired, developed no anxiety or "jumpiness," but felt a strong desire to get
out of the fatiguing situation in which he found himself. This
desire did not show itself, as in the previous case, in a wish to be
killed, but rather in the hope that he might receive wounds
which would incapacitate him from service, for a time at least.

Then he was suddenly buried by a shell. He did not lose
consciousness, but when dug out by his companions he was found
to be deaf and dumb. On his way to the field dressing station
he had a fear of the shells, but this did not persist after his
leaving the zone that was under bombardment.

Physical examination revealed absolutely no abnormality, of
course, to account for his deafness and inability to speak. It
was a purely hysterical condition, and persisted unchanged for
a month. He was then transferred to a hospital for the treatment of functional cases, where he was completely and permanently cured in less than five minutes. This cure was effected
by demonstrating to the patient that he had not really lost his
hearing, the method employed being to make him face a mirror
and observe the start he gave when hands were clapped behind
him. He was spoken to immediately, and told that the jump
he had just given, which he had himself observed in the mirror,

was evidence that he had heard the hand clapping, and that, as his hearing was not lost, neither was his speech. He promptly replied verbally, and had no relapses during the two months before I saw him. All this time he did not suffer from nightmares or from any other anxiety symptoms.

This case is typical of the simple conversion hysteria that develops under the stress of warfare. Not only the history and symptoms are typical, but the speedy and apparently permanent recovery under competent treatment is equally representative of this group.

With these two cases in mind we may proceed to a few general considerations. Officers are affected in the proportion of five to one as compared with privates and non-commissioned officers, although in absolute numbers there are more in the latter group, of course. Explanations for this discrepancy will be offered later. As to the total number of neuroses developing in the different armies, there are no statistics available for general publication. But I have been informed that "shell shock" ranks with what were previously considered the more important conditions (excluding wounds) operating to remove men temporarily or permanently from active service. This makes it at once evident that functional nervous troubles are an extremely important medical problem. Unlike other casualties, however, there is a military significance in the nature of these neuroses. These do not merely cause the removal of many men from active service. As can be easily seen in the first case quoted, there may be the development of a state of fear which may last for weeks or months before the symptoms accumulate sufficiently to incapacitate the soldier totally. No matter how much any man may try to hide his fear, he cannot but unconsciously betray it, and so weaken, or tend to weaken, the morale of his group. This is not merely a psychological deduction, but has been confirmed by the statements of many officers who have observed these cases, and whom I had the opportunity of questioning on the subject.

Another point of military importance is that war neuroses are apparently a corollary of modern methods of fighting. The first reports of these conditions came from the Russo-Japanese war, which would indicate that there is something in the modern trench warfare, combined with the appalling artillery fire, which tends to produce a condition of what might loosely be termed neuropsychic instability. I have had the opportunity of asking several officers who served both in South Africa and in the present war about this matter. The answers are quite consistent. Practically all the officers now in France are familiar with the clinical pictures of the war neuroses, and are therefore competent to say whether they existed in the Boer war or not. None of them observed anything at all similar. It is impossible to consider that the human race can have deteriorated appreciably in a matter of fifteen years, and therefore we are safe in assuming that it is modern warfare which has produced these conditions.

Medical interest in these cases should naturally exceed the interest of the professional soldier. It is the responsibility of the medical corps to treat the sick and prevent diseases from developing. The responsibility of the army medical officer must now, however, go further than this, for the all important discrimination between a definite disease and malingering can be made only by him.

To those who are interested in psychological medicine a new field, and a highly important one, is here opened up. We find in these cases a great simplicity in the psychic mechanisms operating to produce symptoms and the appearance of severe neuroses in people who were apparently absolutely normal before their exposure to the horrors and hardships of this war. We find wishes, fully conscious to the subject, determining symptoms, simple therapeutic measures leading to permanent recovery with astonishing rapidity, and, on the other hand, we see a chronicity of symptoms for which no treatment, or improper treatment, is given.

In all these respects we discover an extraordinary contrast to the phenomena exhibited by neurotics in times of peace. It is therefore reasonable to hope that psycho-pathology can profit greatly by a careful study of the war neuroses. Without minimizing the importance of physical factors, it is safe to say that psychic mechanisms always determine the exact nature of the symptoms.    Physical disabilities, of course, frequently underlie the faulty psychic processes.    We must therefore consider at the outset how our previous psycho-pathological knowledge can be applied to this novel material.    In order to gain our first approach to the problem, account must be taken of what is really, if dispassionately viewed, an extraordinary phenomenon.

At the present time there are millions of men, previously sober, humdrum citizens, with no observable traits of recklessness or bloodthirstiness in their nature, and with a normal interest in their own comfort and security, not only exposing themselves to extraordinary hazards, but cheerfully putting up with extreme discomforts, and engaged in inflicting injuries on fellow human beings, without the repugnance they would have shown in performing similar operations on the bodies of dogs and cats.    It would be impossible to discuss with any completeness the mental mechanisms which result in this astonishing change in character.    It is, however, extremely important to develop some hypothesis, no matter how briefly, to account for this, because one of the phenomena exhibited by the war neuroses is the tendency to return to the mental attitudes of civilian life and to become increasingly obsessed with the horror of warfare.

Deep down in all of us there is, apparently, a primitive instinct that takes a delight in brutality and savagery for themselves alone.    Among civilized peoples these tendencies are, in normal circumstances, quite thoroughly repressed, and gain an outlet, as William James has suggested, only in physical exertions, dangerous exploits and rough and tumble athletic contests.    The origin of this repression is probably to be found in the instinct of gregariousness in the human species, which increases in its power with the advance of civilization, and is necessarily in conflict with all individualistic instincts, whose operation would be inimical to the interests of society.    The repugnance, therefore, of the modern civilized man to cruelty and bloodshed is probably based on the fact that, during centuries of development, the race has frowned upon all lawless individual exhibitions of such tendencies, and that this feeling has become part and parcel of the individual's make-up.

The doctrine of sublimation, as developed by the psychoanalytic school of psychology, furnishes probably the only effective explanation for the lifting of this repression in times of war. A sublimation is an outlet to primitive individualistic instinct, rarely in a direct, more often in a symbolic form, but always so constituted as not to be repugnant to society or to the social instincts of the subject. Any man is not only a member of the human genus, but also, and more immediately, a member of a smaller group, that is, a tribe or a nation. And it is an interesting fact that this group is apt to be more powerful in its influence on the man than is the interest of mankind as a whole. The more primitive is any people, the more does it tend to regard members of other tribes or nations as belonging to a different species, and therefore to be treated as natural enemies, to whom no sympathy or consideration is due. It follows from this that any man's instinctive morality is much more strongly determined by the general standards of the group with which he lives than by any interest in that vaguer conception of mankind as a whole. The average human being is therefore restrained in large measure from the development of his tendencies to lust and cruelty by the innate feeling he enjoys of the deleterious effect such actions would have on his immediate fellows. When war develops, however, a premium is put upon bloodthirstiness, and the community extols the individual who is most effective in inflicting injuries upon the bodies and lives of the members of an opposing group.

This becomes, in effect, a sublimation, for now the soldier can, by the same acts, give vent to his primitive passions and reap the approbation of his fellows. Only two factors may, occasionally, stand in the way of a complete development of this sublimation; the first is the habit of the man's mind, who for years has been educated with ideals of gentleness; the second is that degree of emotional unity, he may possess, that binds him to all mankind, making him sensitive to the sufferings of those outside his group. The combined influence of both these factors is, apparently, insufficient to inhibit an almost universal and fairly free outlet to cruelty in the average modern man, as the present war shows. The soldier is therefore usually able to take delight in the injury he inflicts upon his foe, and to become callously immune to the horrible sights to which he is constantly exposed, since bloodshed, as such, has ceased to be coloured with horror for him.

Another feature in the psychology of war is of clinical importance. Individualistic, and social or herd instincts, are by their very nature in conflict. The predominance of one over the other at any given time depends upon a number of factors, one of the most important of which is the nature of the immediate stimulus. In time of war, either the existence of the tribe or nation is threatened, or there is a possibility of the power of the group being greatly augmented. Either of these possibilities tends to stimulate the social instinct of the individual, rather than his individualistic cravings. Consequently the citizen becomes less of an individual and more an integral part of the society to which he owes allegiance. He thinks less of himself. Greater personal sacrifices become possible, and he is able to feel his reward in the advantages which accrue to his party in the struggle. This gives him the ability to endure fatigue and deprivation, even cheerfully to face death itself, in a way that would be quite impossible in times of peace. This and the enjoyment of bloodshed probably constitute the two most important factors in the production of the change of character which the civilian undergoes in becoming a soldier[1].

In recent years, those who have been interested in the more minute psychological study of neuroses, particularly those of the psycho-analytic school, have found that before the onset of actual symptoms, there is apt to be a period during which there are changes in the patient's activities or outlook upon life. Very often these changes are the result of environmental accident, but, whether coming from within or without, they consist essentially in a change of his adaptation to the situation in which

[1] For fuller discussion of this topic, see J. T. MacCurdy, *The Psychology of War*, Heinemann, London, 1917.

he is placed, and involve a loss or weakness of sublimations which he has previously enjoyed. A knowledge of this phenomenon is of considerable aid in studying war neuroses, because we find that an analogous change takes place in the adaptation of the soldier to his task before the appearance of active symptoms. Anyone, who is at all familiar with the phenomena of modern trench warfare, can see that it makes a great demand on the devotion of the belligerents and offers little personal satisfaction in return. In previous wars the soldiers, it is true, were called upon to suffer fatigue and expose themselves to great danger. In return, however, they were compensated by the excitement of more active operations, the more frequent possibility of gaining some satisfaction in active hand to hand fighting, where they might feel the joy of personal prowess. Now, the soldier must remain for days, weeks, even months, in a narrow trench or a stuffy dugout, exposed to a constant danger of the most fearful kind; namely, bombardment with high explosive shells, which come from some unseen source, and against which no personal agility or wit is of any avail. This naturally occasions great fatigue, and, on the other hand, opportunities of active hand to hand fighting are rare, so that a man may be exposed for months to the appalling effects of bombardment and never once have a chance to retaliate in a personal way. Consequently the sublimations described above are more difficult to maintain than in any previous war. The soldier becomes fatigued (developing symptoms which will be discussed later) and not unnaturally finds it difficult to remain satisfied with his situation. His adaptation to warfare is, therefore, soon weakened or lost. His disregard of the carnage and death around him is gone, and he becomes every day more acutely sensitive to the horrors which surround him. This sensitiveness may develop even to the point of pity for the foe, which is naturally an emotion most incapacitating for a soldier.

With this dislike for the war there is inevitably some degree of resentment at the State which has sent him to fight, although this is apt to come only vaguely into full consciousness. The bonds uniting him to the common cause are definitely loosened, however, and as a consequence his individual feelings begin to assert themselves. Accidents to which he was previously liable, but to which he was indifferent, are now viewed with apprehension. He becomes fearful of the dangers opposing him, so that his courage is no longer automatic but forced. According as he has high or low ideals, is more or less intelligent, he feels a shame before his fellows as a coward, or feels ill-treated by his superiors in being forced to continue fighting. His feeling of cowardice may lead to superhuman efforts of self-control, but these lead only to a cumulative increase of his fatigue. Naturally he grows mentally and nervously more and more unstable, but is prevented from leaving the line, either by his superior officers or by his own shame at the thought of "going sick," which is frequently looked upon as a sign of weakness. Those of lesser intelligence often regard their terrors as indications of approaching insanity, and thus another worry is added to the strains under which they suffer. Once a man has acquired this unhappy condition any trifling accident, such as a mild concussion from an exploding shell, or some particularly unpleasant experience, may cause a final break and lead to such an exaggeration of symptoms already present that he becomes totally incompetent.

It is not unnatural that anyone in this situation should look for some relief, and, unconsciously at least, this must be a powerful factor in the production of disabling symptoms. In many cases, after more or less of these prodromal difficulties, symptoms appear that seem to be specifically directed against the man's capacity to fight.

As many physicians in England, previously apathetic or antagonistic to psycho-analysis, now admit, the general mechanisms of repression of emotionally toned ideas with their reappearance when repression fails, are responsible for the production of the symptoms of war neuroses. Psycho-analysts in civilian practice claim that the individualistic tendencies in question are preponderantly related to the sex instinct. In war, however, this does not seem to be the case, these latter tendencies coming into play, apparently, only as a complication. The reason for this is probably to be found in the fact that in warfare

the instincts of self-interest and self-preservation, which are just
as primitive and basic as the sex instinct, are involved in a way
that they never are in normal civilian life. The psychological
factors are consequently much more simple, and it may be that
this explains the extraordinary amenability of the war neuroses
to treatment. Personality studies of many of the cases, however,
show a previous weakness in adaptability that is confined to
such demands as are essentially related to sex. These individuals, although they may never manifest symptoms directly related to any erotic tendencies, are nevertheless apt to suffer
sooner or more severely than their completely normal fellows.
The explanation for these two phenomena is perhaps to be found
in the fact that sex adaptation is quite the most difficult of all
those which the individual has to make in modern civilization.
The same fundamental weakness exhibits itself in his failure to
respond fully to the most trying demands of civilian life, namely,
those of sex adaptation, and in his inability to meet the demands
of war. In other words, the neurotic in times of peace may have
his symptoms on account of poor adaptation in the sex sphere,
but this is fundamentally dependent on some vague constitutional defect from which he suffers. It is this defect which also
makes him liable to lose his efficiency in the unparalleled strain
of modern war. One makes inquiry into a patient's past life,
therefore, not only in order to discover what there may have
been in his previous character which would directly affect his
capacity as a soldier, but also to gain some rough idea of how
resistant he had previously been to the most disturbing influences of life.

# CHAPTER III

## ANXIETY STATES

THE term "Anxiety States" is chosen to designate one of the two clinical groups into which the war neuroses fall, for the reason that anxiety is the most prominent and consistent feature in the clinical picture. These cases bear most resemblance to what is frequently termed "neurasthenia" in civil practice, but it is thought better to avoid this term in the present instance on account of the vagueness which almost universally exists as to what neurasthenia is. Unfortunately the term has been used to include practically every neurosis.

The *clinical course* of an anxiety state is as follows: the patient is a man who may or may not have had a past history of abnormality. The existence of abnormality affects the clinical course of his neurosis in that it is apt to indicate an earlier onset, more marked symptoms and a longer duration. But there are too many exceptions to this statement to make it more than a generalization.

When the civilian enlists or is commissioned, he at once enters into a totally new life, and, provided he is a tolerably normal individual, quickly adapts himself to it. This is demonstrated by his eagerness to learn his new duties, his pleasure in his accomplishment as training progresses, and in an increased sociability. It is frequently found that an individual who has been rather shy will make more friends after entering the army than he ever did before. It is, of course, unneeessary to state that training almost invariably has a marked effect on physique in the direction of improvement.

The mental attitude of the new soldier on leaving for the front is of some interest. The majority of men are eager for their new experiences and look forward to active service without much apprehension. A few, however, of the more introspective type, are unable to keep their thoughts away from wounds and death; some with a distinct fear of failure, that is, a fear that their courage may not be equal to the demands made upon it. With occasional men this apprehension is sufficient to precipitate a neurosis, but the clinical features of this are more apt to resemble the peace, than the war, type, and none are included in this report. It is important to note that some momentary disquietude at this stage is not necessarily indicative of coming failure. There are men who approach the actual battlefield with considerable misgiving, but are surprised to find how quickly they become indifferent to the dangers they meet there.

The first actual trial which the recruit usually meets is the experience of being shelled. Naturally the intensity of the bombardment varies greatly, and if the shells are falling at long intervals of time and at considerable distance, it is only the most unstable who are particularly affected. Few, if any, as far as one can learn, are absolutely normal on introduction to a heavy bombardment. By far the commonest response is one of fear, usually accompanied with the idea of running away, which the subject himself sees to be absurd. Although the men may make an effort to hide the signs of this fear, they are so frequently evident under initial shelling that the military authorities count on their appearance. Their presence at this time is no indication of the degree of indifference which may later develop. A less common reaction is that of excitement, accompanied even with a kind of spurious elation. The man has a tendency to make facetious remarks about the shells, to laugh at feeble witticisms, and very often feels under considerable motor tension, there being a pressing desire to do something, to do it immediately and do it hard. A still more unusual but very interesting reaction is that of slowness or languor (which may succeed primary fear). This may be accompanied by a depressive affect or by lethargy so extreme that the individual will lie down and go perforce to sleep with a pathological indifference to the danger.

None of these reactions seem, of themselves, to be indicative of the future adaptability of the soldier. That is determined much more by the duration of these symptoms. Most men recover quite soon (a matter of a day or so) and then become indifferent to the possibility of being hit, and capable of philosophically considering the chances. This development is usually accompanied by, or is the result of, learning to recognize the location and direction of the shells by the sound they make in travelling through the air. When a man can tell from the sound that a shell is travelling some distance over his head and will fall a hundred yards to the rear, that sound has no further terrifying effect on him.

If the primary bombardment be sufficiently heavy, the soldier sees his first casualties, and it is a rare man who is not struck with horror at the sight of the mangled remains of his comrades. The man who is going to make a good soldier, however, quickly becomes accustomed to this. Similarly, there may be an initial inhibition with horror at the thought of inflicting wounds on, or killing, an opponent, but this, too, is a temporary phase. Individuals who cannot recover fully from their initial fear, horror, or reluctance to inflict injury, never build up that sublimation which we have described, and so are poorly adapted to a soldier's life. These men are very quickly fatigued and develop disabling symptoms.

The first sign of an approaching neurosis is fatigue. The word sign, rather than symptom, is used because fatigue as such is a condition which is completely removed by rest, and rest of quite brief duration. For the neurosis, fatigue is of importance, as it is the almost universal occasion of the dissatisfaction with his work which leads to a breaking down of the soldier's adaptation and the development of more permanent symptoms. The conditions producing fatigue are both physical and mental. Those on the physical side are the obvious ones of long hours of duty, combined often with irregularity of meals, shortness of water, exposure to extremes of temperature, constant wetting, etc. Although these factors need no detailed consideration on account of their obviousness, their importance in producing fatigue cannot be too strongly emphasized. Important as they are, however, they are probably of less influence in the production of neurotic fatigue than are the purely mental influences. The most common and important of these is the strain of continuing in a dull routine that demands a constant alertness, a speediness of decision, complete self-confidence and a spontaneous eagerness. And this mental attitude must be maintained hours, even days, on end, without sleep, often without the distraction of food, and in the face of constant danger. Other, more personal, factors contribute to the development of fatigue. A man, for instance, may be placed under the authority of some one who is antagonistic to him and makes everything as difficult as possible. This naturally leads to distrust, and once a man's confidence is lost in his superiors it is soon impossible for him to disregard the strain under which he suffers. Many men, too, have peculiarities that make them susceptible to particular discomforts. Such things as the presence of vermin, and the frequency of bad odours, particularly where there are many unburied bodies, are factors of no mean importance in slowly disheartening the soldier. In fact, one can safely say that in view of the many external physical difficulties, a soldier can be kept in the best mental condition only when he is not irritated by things which affect his special sensibilities, and, most important, when he feels socially comfortable with his mates. Not infrequently the death of a close friend or comrade may be the signal for the stress of warfare to make its effects known.

The above views present this neuro-psychic fatigue as a product of environmental, or of mental, factors. It must be mentioned, however, that other views are held on this matter. When these patients are finally brought to a hospital, it is often found that they have a low blood-pressure. Temporary symptoms indicative of thyroid disturbance are also seen not infrequently. Some students of "shell shock" have therefore made the claim that the fundamental and primary cause of the neuroses lies in the ductless glands. They consider that the patients have succumbed to the strain of warfare because their endocrinic functions were less stable than those of their fellows. Considering that the vast bulk of these men have never shown any symptoms earlier in their lives of internal secretion disease, this is probably too sweeping a statement to be accepted as such. It must be borne in mind, however, that some chemical change is probably present in neuro-psychic fatigue. The poison—whatever it is that affects the central nervous system—may easily be the product of some endocrinic reaction to abnormal conditions. This opens up an important and not unpromising field for research. Civilian life does not favour the development of fatigue to anything like the same extent as does the stress of war. Consequently, any chemical changes must be present in a greater degree than in the milder states of mere "tiredness" which we meet in times of peace. We might therefore hope that what has heretofore remained undiscovered, might now be found to the immense benefit of neuro-pathology.

It can readily be seen that the more in the mental sphere a man's responsibilities lie, the more quickly will he be affected, and it is a striking fact that anxiety conditions in the pure state occur almost exclusively among officers. It is their task, not merely to keep their own feelings in subjugation, but to inspire the men beneath them with courage and enthusiasm.

The evidences of fatigue are almost exclusively in the mental sphere. It goes without saying that there is a subjective feeling of weariness. This, however, is so common and so easily produced that it is of no especial significance. What one can term fatigue in a clinical sense appears when other symptoms develop. These are a feeling of tenseness, a restless desire for action or distraction, irritability, difficulty in concentration, and a tendency to start at any sudden sound (without fear), the sound being usually that of exploding shells. This reaction of nervous starting is so common that it is universally known by the officers and men as "jumpiness." There is usually a slight improvement in the feeling of weariness toward night, as a certain degree of excitement accumulates which enables the individual to disregard his difficulties.

The nocturnal symptoms are even more distinctive. There is great difficulty in getting to sleep, with a long period of hypnagogic hallucinations. Whatever has been the dominating experience of the day appears in troublesome vision before the eyes of the soldier, who although knowing that what he sees is not actually there, is still unable either to go to sleep or to awaken himself sufficiently to banish the visions. The only emotional reaction is a feeling of irritation with restlessness. Fatigue as such does not seem to produce fear. When sleep does come, it is often troubled by repeated dreams of the occupational type where the soldier is trying to do whatever was his task during the day, is having constant difficulty and meeting with no success in accomplishment. The sleep, too, is frequently interrupted by the man suddenly awakening with a jump, although he is not conscious of this waking being the result of any incident in his previous dream. As a result, he gets many less hours sleep than he expected, and little benefit from the sleep he does achieve. He awakes in the morning more tired than when he lay down, feeling slow and unwilling to assume the duties to which he has to force himself.

When this situation has continued for some time and become cumulatively worse, fear, as has been said, develops, and also horror of the sights around him. Both of these are signs that the "war sublimation" has failed. The soldier finds himself, when alone and not mentally occupied with his duty, thinking of the horrible sights he has seen. He dwells obsessively on the difficulties which surround him, on the frictions he may have with brother or superior officers, and cannot keep his mind away from the possibility of injury. It is interesting to note that the British soldiers are singularly free, at this stage, from homesickness, although the Canadian troops are very liable to it. This is presumably the result of the longer distance from home of the latter and the impossibility of return within the near future.

A man in this condition is very apt to find a certain externalization of his difficulty in thinking about war in general, and there are probably no more fervid pacifists in existence than many of the men who are conscientiously fighting day after day. Many of them acquire with their reluctance to bloodshed such a pity for the enemy that they find it difficult to fight effectively.

At this stage when fear is developing, a man begins to lose his judgment concerning the direction of shells. At first, he feels frightened when he hears the shell coming, although he knows it is not going to land where he is. Later, he loses the ability to gauge its direction, and consequently every shell seems aimed at him personally. Naturally in such a situation a heavy bombardment becomes almost intolerable. It is necessary, however, particularly for the officer, that all signs of fear should be hidden, and to his other difficulties is added the fear that he may not be able to hide his fear—another factor in the vicious circle.

Thus afflicted, the soldier now has ideas of escape, the nature of which has considerable influence on the symptoms to follow. There are three practicable avenues of escape; the man may receive an incapacitating wound, he may be taken prisoner, or he may be killed. One who manifests an anxiety state is always one with high ideals of his duty. We find, therefore, that none of them entertain the hope of disabling wounds. Nor do they consciously seek surrender, but it is interesting that they not infrequently dream of it at this stage. The third possibility is the most alluring, as it offers complete release and is quite compatible with all standards of duty. It is not unnatural, therefore, that many of these unfortunates who are constantly obsessed with fear perform most reckless acts. Almost universally there are thoughts of suicide, and many of the men thus afflicted will plan different methods of accomplishing their own deaths in ways which could not be subsequently regarded as suicidal.

When once the desire for death has become fixed, a complete breakdown is imminent. This breakdown, as a rule, occurs after some accident, which is either physical or mental. The commonest physical accident is the exposure to the explosion of a shell, which either produces a brief unconsciousness by concussion, or, possibly, poisons the individual with some noxious gas. After this accident, the neurosis is suddenly established in an incapacitating form, or if the fatigue symptoms have just begun, they suddenly become very much worse.

The mental accidents should properly be called precipitating factors. They consist of psychic traumata such as particularly horrible sights, the mangling of some close friend, or the killing of all others in the immediate environment. Occasionally it is an extremely dangerous situation, such as arises when a company is isolated in an advanced trench and subjected to a pitilessly methodical bombardment that seems certain to kill every occupant of the trench sooner or later. A very frequent occurrence is burial with earth thrown up by an exploding shell. Some clinicians are inclined to attribute all the results of such burial to concussion, whereas a thorough examination of many patients who have been buried reveals the fact that there have been no symptoms developed which could not be fully accounted for on the basis of mental shock, and, on the other hand, that there have been none that point definitely to concussion. It is important to note that this quite frequent accident produces little or no effect on the normal individual, but is extremely trying, if not actually incapacitating to the soldier who has begun to manifest symptoms.

Another precipitating factor, that is obviously purely mental, is the disappointment ensuing on a refusal of "leave" from the trenches when that has been expected. The man whose ability to continue fighting has been put to a great strain, is enabled to keep going by the thought that there is a definite end in view. When this end is suddenly and indefinitely postponed, his last remaining source of encouragement is gone and he collapses. Similarly, when the soldier is sent back to a rest camp for a short stay and this has proved insufficient to restore his equilibrium, the order to return to the front line may cause the sudden development of incapacitating symptoms.

It is both theoretically and practically of the first importance to recognize that actual wounding does not disable the soldier neurotically, no matter what his mental and nervous condition may be. This is really not difficult to understand. As we have seen, the man has an urgent desire to escape from an intolerable situation, and a large part of the motivation of the symptoms comes directly from this wish. A wound is obviously an ideal form of relief. So true is this that it is said to be a common occurrence for a soldier who has had a foot or a leg blown off, to dance about on the remaining one shouting with joy that he has got a "Blighty one" (Blighty being the Tommies' slang for England; that is, a wound which will take him home).

The acute symptoms of the neurosis may be ushered in with a stuporous state. As I have said before, I have not had an opportunity of examining cases at this stage, and so must rely on what can be gained from the patients' own retrospects, and what is to be learned from others. It seems that these stuporous states that ensue suddenly after concussion or some mental trauma are of two types, organic and functional, although the latter may slowly emerge from the former. The organic type is marked by a true loss of consciousness, followed by a period during which consciousness reappears and can be maintained for a short time, only to lapse again. This "dipping" may endure for days, even weeks. While conscious, the patient is extremely confused, disoriented, usually complains of violent headache, is frequently incontinent and may have to be catheterized. A delirium is very frequent, the content of which is constant aggression on the part of the enemy, either with bayonets, bombs or shells, against which the patient is largely or completely powerless.

The functional type of stuporous state may be ushered in by a condition which apparently expresses the acme of fear, the patient lying with dilated pupils, in a cold sweat, with shallow breathing, incapable of any voluntary movement, and often trembling violently. Following this, there is a phase when voluntary movement is possible, during which he is dazed, inactive, confused and amnesic, and may use gestures in place of speech. Myers thinks that the "unconsciousness" of which so many patients subsequently tell may really be this stuporous state. Unfortunately he attempts no discrimination between organic and functional symptoms in these conditions.

While still in a stuporous state, the patient may suffer from hallucinations concerning which he is amnesic or confused later. It is only the more severe cases, of course, which show marked or prolonged symptoms of stupor. In others, the hypnagogic hallucinations of which we have spoken pass over into somewhat similar visions, which are now accompanied by fear. That is, in place of a repetition of the day's work, in the visions on going to sleep, the patient sees soldiers advancing against him with bayonets, throwing bombs at him, feels mines exploding beneath his feet, or he hears shells coming shrieking toward him. Insight as to the reality of these visions varies. Occasionally it is constant. More often it is applied with some effort on the part of the patient, whereas it is quite unusual for it to be consistently absent. Any sudden sound, such as a door slamming, is interpreted as the explosion of a shell, with consequent terror. The patient jumps with fright, although he usually realizes very quickly the real nature of the sound.

In his preliminary symptoms, the patient, as a rule, may have been bothered with dreams of the occupational type, but has had few, if any, nightmares. Once the neurosis reaches this acute stage, however, sleep becomes torture owing to the violence of nightmares. These, like the hallucinations, have a purely war content, the setting of which is, as a rule, the section of the line in which the patient has last been, or that section in which he may have been subjected to most severe strain. The exact nature of the injuries which seem imminent in the dreams, naturally varies with the type of fighting in which the man has been engaged. The enemy is throwing bombs at him, which explode at his feet, he is about to be bayoneted, he is shot down in an aeroplane or shells are raining upon him. Unlike dreams in times of peace, no amount of cross-questioning can produce any details which would indicate that there is any inaccuracy in the delineation of the normal environment. That is, the soldier is always in France, he is always in a trench, his comrades are always his natural comrades, nothing is distorted except that he is invariably powerless to retaliate, and his fear is infinitely greater than it ever is while he is awake in a situation at all similar. This last point is quite interesting psychologically. Patients who have these dreams while still in the trenches may be completely paralyzed with fear in their dreams, and yet be capable of performing their duties during the day with few signs of nervousness; occasionally they are even totally free from fear during the day.

The patient is, of course, awakened, as in the civilian night-mares, in a cold sweat of terror; frequently he awakes screaming. As even a few minutes' sleep means the appearance of such a nightmare, there is added to his previous difficulty in falling to sleep, a fear of sleep, and this reduces his actual rest, obtained without sedatives, to a very small amount. In fact, patients may go for some weeks getting only a few minutes' actual normal sleep any night.

Naturally then, the fatigue from which he previously suffered is greatly increased. It is particularly in evidence in the morning, improving somewhat as the day goes on, and apt to be much worse again by night. Blood-pressure may be quite low according to some observers. Some have found this so regularly, and have seen it rise again so consistently with improvement, that they have concluded that there is a primary disturbance in the glands of internal secretion. It is not unlikely that a change in endocrinic functions determines the low pressure, but the evidence seems to point toward this change being secondary to fatigue (or concussion). It must be borne in mind that the degree of fatigue developed in active warfare is incomparably greater than anything we ever see in times of peace, and that a low blood-pressure is therefore to be expected. Patients in the acute phases of the neurosis are frequently subjected to photophobia. Tremors are, I believe, always present. These occur most frequently in the hands and arms, but may appear in any part of the body. They are present both at rest and on voluntary movement, the latter being much more marked. There is also sometimes a slight ataxia which is never really disabling. Both tremors and ataxia are prone to be much exaggerated when attention is directed to them. Cyanosis of the hands and feet is frequently observed, but perhaps not more often than in soldiers who have no neurosis, but have been exposed to the inclemencies of the weather during many winter months.

Symptoms suggestive of disturbance of the thyroid gland are very frequent, but usually of short duration. The eyes protrude slightly, and the upper eyelid may lag behind the eyeball on looking downward; the pulse is rapid, excessive sweating is extremely common, and sometimes there is a slight enlargement of the thyroid gland. Headaches, rarely of extreme violence, are common.

Objective mental symptoms are shown occasionally by tics, such as blinking the eyes, or a grimace accompanied by a withdrawal of the head, suggesting the starting back from something unpleasant.

Histories of these patients sometimes state that they have been subject to hysterical "fits," so that epilepsy has been considered. Although unable to observe any of these attacks myself, I have carefully questioned a number of patients who have had them, and from their account I should be inclined to believe that they were not convulsions, in any sense of the word, but much more like tantrum reactions, and similar to the performances of a child who lies on the floor and kicks when particularly upset.

The facial expression of many anxiety cases is sufficiently typical for a diagnosis to be made by mere inspection. The face is drawn, showing signs of fatigue, while the emotional strain is exhibited by chronic frowning with considerable wrinkling of the forehead. The patients look as if they were under great strain, and maintaining control of themselves with effort. The expression suggests a chronic mental, rather than physical, pain.

As most of these patients are kept in bed for some time, they are apt to be weak on getting up, and as a result find themselves unsteady on their feet when they attempt to walk. As a rule, this is recovered from quite quickly. Occasionally, however, the staggering, uncertain gait with coarse tremors of the feet and legs, which is natural to a weakened patient, becomes with all the symptoms exaggerated, a chronic gait. This is rare in officers but more common among privates.

There is an interesting feature of the mental state of these patients, not at all obvious, but subjectively painful, and one that has considerable effect on the course of the disease when it is well marked. As has been said, these men, while still in the firing line, are apt to think more of themselves than they previously had thought, and consequently to get out of touch with their fellows. This latter tendency is almost universally present when the neurosis is firmly established. The patient suffers considerably from a lack of sociability, and of spontaneous affection. This is probably due, in part, to a sense of unworthiness which develops with a feeling of cowardice. As in almost any neurosis, there is considerable introversion. Many a patient wants to be alone, and, although he is always capable of making a good impression socially in a formal way, he finds it difficult to exhibit any signs of affection. The man who is visited by his mother, his wife, or his sweetheart is a disappointment both to himself and to his visitor in that it is impossible for him to give any convincing proof of his affection. This finds expression physically in a painfully obvious way through the symptom of impotence, which is, so far as I have been able to learn, universally present in the anxiety state, either as such or in the form of its equivalent, lack of erotic feeling. Even in quite mild cases it occurs, and its demonstration may be a distinct shock to the patient. More frequently no attempt at intercourse is made, through lack of desire.

These symptoms continue acutely for a few weeks in most cases, sometimes for months in the more severe neuroses. All the more obvious symptoms tend to abate gradually without particularly painstaking treatment. The dreams grow less frequent, and usually disappear. Quite frequently the content changes when the patient has been away from the trenches for some time. Distortions occur whereby the setting comes to include more of the normal peace environment. For example, the patient may begin to have normal dreams of civilian life which will be suddenly interrupted by the appearance of the enemy with bombs or bayonets. A man may be playing golf, when the foe suddenly appears on the green. A very interesting change of content occurs occasionally and marks a radical emotional change. For some time dreams will proceed, in which the enemy is invariably successful and the dreamer powerless. Then the dreamer begins to show fight, and for some nights may struggle, although still defeated. Next, the battle becomes a draw. Finally, the dreamer begins to get the upper hand and is able to enjoy the

fight of which he dreams, because he invariably punishes the
enemy. Such a sequence augurs well, of course, for the man's
further adaptability in the firing line. When improvement
begins, the fatigue lessens sufficiently for the patient to leave
his bed and indulge in mild activities about the hospital. He is
surprised, however, to find how quickly he becomes tired, even
exhausted, when he goes through the streets, or attempts to
play some game. But, unless there are other complications,
this phase of fatigability, rather than chronic fatigue, is quickly
passed.

The constant apprehensiveness which persists throughout the
day in the acute stages, disappears, but in its place there remains a good deal of "jumpiness." In the earlier stages a
sudden noise is interpreted as an explosion. Then the real
nature of the sound is instantaneously recognized, but the
patient is frightened, which suggests that unconsciously the
sound is still regarded as a shell. Later the habit of starting at
any sound persists without any fear. That this may be purely
a neurotic habit, is demonstrated by such instances as the following: I was talking to a patient when he moved to knock some
ashes from a cigarette into a small bowl. While his hand was
approaching the bowl, a door slammed. The patient proceeded
to execute his movement quite carefully and then to jump
violently, although more than a second had elapsed between the
sound and the jump. At this stage the patient can, if he exerts
sufficient effort, train himself to remain calm when sudden
noises occur. Quite frequently the patients who are more intelligent can remember accurately the phases of development
and disappearance of this symptom.

The patient has now come to appear objectively normal, but
grave defects are still subjectively present to interfere with his
renewed adaptation to trench warfare. He finds, for instance,
that crowded traffic makes him excessively nervous. He is fearful that his taxicab will run over some one in the street, or that
there will be collisions. He finds himself dizzy if he is in a high
place, or looks out of a window some distance from the ground.
He cannot enter a tunnel, and thunder-storms terrify him. Per-

haps his most distressing symptom is his feeling of incompetence and his lack of desire to return to the front. He is a subject of serious mental conflict. He knows that duty calls him to fight again, and that he ought cheerfully to assume these duties, but he recognizes that he is a coward, feels great shame over this, and is even more ashamed of the lack of desire to do his bit. It is this final phase which may be indefinitely prolonged if appropriate psychological treatment is not available.

When acute symptoms subside, complications are prone to appear. It would not be surprising to anyone familiar with the psychology of the neurotic to learn that the disappearance of obviously incapacitating symptoms may be the signal for others to develop which would make return to the front impossible. Naturally, these complications occur mainly, if not exclusively, in those who have before the war been not quite normal. A man, for instance, who has previously had a neurosis, may produce his old symptoms again. Captain Rivers[1] thinks that adaptation to war demands a repression of all neurotic tendencies and abnormalities, which, on account of this repression, increase in intensity, and therefore reappear with unwonted strength when the patient has been absent from the front for some time.

A frequent complication is depression. This rarely, if ever, reaches the point of retardation. It is much more a subjective feeling of hopelessness and shame for incompetence and cowardice. Sometimes the depression is the accompaniment of obsessing thoughts about the horrors the patient has seen, and about the horrors of war in general. Very often he is depressed because he feels that he is not being treated well. This last is probably a development of the lack of contact with his fellows which has been previously enjoyed. The patient, having become interested more in his own welfare than in the needs of the army or the country, is prone to dwell on the sacrifices he has made and the obligations of the State to him. Such patients are therefore morbidly interested in having attention paid to them. This is somewhat different from ordinary hypochondria, in that it is

---

[1] Personal communication.

not a physical symptom for which the patient demands attention so much as it is himself, his personality, which he feels to be neglected.

The diagnosis of this neurosis naturally offers very little difficulty. The only condition with which it could be confused is malingering. The history and appearance of these patients should, however, never leave much doubt in the mind of the physician. Some history of slow onset and gradual dissatisfaction is invariably present in those cases who do not break down after physical trauma. Even those who have suffered from severe concussion will give a similar history, although it may be reduced to the presence of mild symptoms for a short time before the accident. I was unable to find a single sufferer from pure anxiety who did not give a history of some prodromal difficulties. The concussion cases also show signs of organic disturbance of the brain function which are diagnostic (dipping of consciousness, confusion, disorientation, etc.). The malingerer is not likely to speak frankly about his gradually increasing terror, whereas the man suffering from a true anxiety neurosis is, as a rule, extraordinarily open and frank about the matter. The appearance, too, of drawn face, staring eyes, exhibiting obvious distress, combined with a rapid pulse and excessive sweating, is something which it would be very hard to imitate consciously. Difficulty in eliminating malingering occurs almost exclusively with the conversion hysterias rather than with the anxiety neuroses.

We must next consider in somewhat more detail, and with illustrative cases, the various factors of importance in the production of the anxiety state.

# CHAPTER IV

## MENTAL MAKE-UP

THERE are certain features in the personality study which are more or less directly related to the capacity of the individual for warfare. It goes without saying that one always makes inquiries as to the existence of actual nervous breakdowns. An individual who has once given way to a neurosis is obviously more likely to be unstable than one who has not. What one may term neurotic tendencies rather than neuroses must be searched for diligently. The man who, as a child, has suffered from night terrors and fear of the dark will probably, under a strain, be more apt to become fearful than one who has not. Similarly an individual who has been either chronically, or as a child, afraid of thunder-storms, is apt to be affected more quickly by shell fire, as the noise of bombardment is extremely like that of a violent thunder-storm. A man with a tendency to claustrophobia, which in times of peace may be indicated only by a slight feeling of faintness in an underground train, or by an unusual sensitiveness to the bad air in such a situation, or a mild feeling of discomfort, is apt to be fearful of dugouts being blown in, or to be particularly afraid that he may be buried by a shell. The existence of such claustrophobic tendencies may be determined by questioning as to symptoms of all kinds while in a subway, or by finding out whether the patient has suffered from nightmares of premature burial, or of being enclosed in some small space. Great sensitiveness to cruelty, horror of bloodshed and accidents, discomfort at the sight of animals being killed, unusual sensitiveness to pain, either in himself or others, are all indications of more than normal difficulty which the soldier may have in accustoming himself to the horrors of war. Occasionally this abnormality may be expressed in a morbid fascination for the horrible.

Seclusiveness, as has been said, is important in that it is an indication of general lack of adaptability, and is, of course, more likely to occur in an individual who is not quite up to par in his ability to meet any situation, particularly one such as war, that demands the highest degree of normality. It has, however, another and more direct importance. The soldier who is not naturally sociable has, as a consequence, less of an outlet for his feelings in the trenches, and is less distracted from the thoughts of the painfulness of his situation than is his normal companion. As a result, he becomes more quickly a prey to all the influences that generate fatigue and dissatisfaction.

The following cases exhibit different types of make-up and the effect of previous abnormalities on the development and symptoms of anxiety neuroses.

CASE III. The patient is a lieutenant, of 25, an artist before he joined the army, who had never had any nervous breakdown, but with the rather high-strung sensitive disposition frequently found in those who adopt this profession. As a child he had frequent night terrors, which disappeared as he grew older, but evidently had made quite an impression on him. In fact he spoke of the dreams which developed in his neurosis as a return of his childish nightmares. He never was able to prevent giddiness when he was in an especially high place, but had no fear of thunder-storms. He was abnormally sensitive to the sight of blood, and more sympathetic than is usual. He had no dreams of premature burial, but as a child remembers having fear of being shut up in a small place. In his adult life he had an uncomfortable apprehensiveness when on the underground railway, and was positively terrified by the "switchback"—a railway in amusement parks that dashes suddenly into sepulchral caverns.

All his life he was of a rather retiring and self-conscious disposition, but constantly struggled against it, and was able to make fair adaptations. For example, he played the usual games at school, and creditably, too, but never was capable of abandoning his self-consciousness and joining in with the usual boyish

pranks with any great enthusiasm.  He was similarly rather shy
with girls, but did not let this prevent him from going out in
society, although he had no puppy love affairs.  He fell in love
with only one girl and married her immediately before entering
the army.  As practically all of his married life had been spent
away from home, it was impossible to see how well he would have
adapted himself to marriage.

He reacted well to his training and became more sociable and
self-reliant.  When he arrived in France and came under shell
fire he was frightened, and although he recovered to a certain
extent from his initial terror, he never was capable of wholly
ridding himself from fear of shells.

The horrors of war made a constant impression upon him, and
afflicted his sensitive nature to such an extent that he never
could bring himself to enjoy the fight.  The best that he could do
was to be unaware, in an advance, that he was killing men.  He
was not afraid of machine guns, had some slight fears of snipers,
but found a constant strain in waiting in the trenches for shells
to come, the likelihood of which was always in his mind.  His
claustrophobic tendencies appeared in that he was afraid of the
dugouts and hated to go into them, although they offered the
only protection from bombardment.  He always felt that a shell
might come and block the entrance so that he would be buried
alive.  He never dreamed of this, however.

This man was obviously not adapted for any continued stretch
of fighting, and as a result, within a couple of months of reaching
the front he began to show symptoms of fatigue in sleeplessness,
hypnagogic hallucinations, and a good deal of "jumpiness" in
the daytime.  Fear quickly appeared, and then his condition
got rapidly worse.  Being a man of high ideals as to his duty, he
made great efforts to keep all signs of fear from his men, and to
appear absolutely intrepid before them.  In this he succeeded,
but only to produce such a strain that he felt after a few weeks
that it was only a matter of time before he would have to give
up.  While in this condition, a shell dropped one day on the
parados and threw enough dirt into the trench where he was
standing to cover his legs up to the knees.  He became absolutely

terrified, although physically he felt no effects whatever, did not lose consciousness nor become at all confused. It seems not unlikely that this accident, which was a small enough affair in the light of his daily experiences, represented symbolic burial. At any rate, whatever its psychological significance, he became completely unstrung and felt that it was absolutely impossible to continue his duties. He therefore reported sick, and the medical officer, observing his condition, sent him to the hospital. That night he dreamed that he was taken prisoner by the Germans, and had to confess, when he related his dream, that with it there was a certain feeling of relief in that he was by this event free from all responsibilities of "carrying on." He never had had this idea during the daytime, however, so far as he could remember, but had only wished for death.

The day following this dream, he felt still worse, more fearful than before (although he was out of danger) and extremely sensitive to noises. That night terrifying dreams began. These were always of some untoward event, the most frequent of which was that the enemy would penetrate his trench, and rush at him, with bayonets, one of which was just about to pierce his chest when he would awake in an agony of terror. He said that in these dreams he always wanted to scream with fright, which was an idea which would never occur to him in the daytime in the trenches, no matter how frightened he might be.

When he first went into the trenches he had occasional emissions during sleep. Once his symptoms began, these ceased, and he had no erotic thoughts whatever. The latter did not return until he was nearly recovered from his neurosis.

After about three weeks the dreams began to lessen in their frequency, although the content changed not at all. Finally they disappeared. When they had been absent for about a week, he dreamed one night that he was being tied down by some soldiers on a stretcher, for what purpose he did not know, but he was very much frightened and was trying to scream when he awoke. This, of course, was not related directly to any actual experience at the front, and it remained an isolated dream.

Physically he showed some fatigability when I examined him

about three weeks after leaving the front. He had prominent eyes, a rapid pulse and some sweating. His tremors were not marked, and did not endure for long. His was a case where a few weeks' rest in bed, without other treatment, caused all the obvious symptoms to disappear. None of them, in fact, had ever been particularly severe, except the dreams, and of these he had never had more than one or two in any one night.

This history is rather typical of the patient who is poorly adapted to fighting. The struggle begins at the first moment of entering the trenches, and the mental difficulties increase out of all proportion to the physical fatigue. As a result, these patients are apt to give up before they have struggled long enough against their symptoms to exhaust seriously their fund of nervous energy. The symptoms, therefore, do not become so intense, nor do they last so long as they do with those who are normal enough to become well adapted to the fighting and then spend weeks and even months in a strenuous effort to fight their symptoms after the "break in compensation" has set in.

To get such a patient as this back to the firing line, is, of course, a good deal more of a problem than to relieve him of his acute symptoms.

CASE IV. The patient is a lieutenant in the artillery, 23 years of age. He was always high-strung and sensitive, and thinks that he would have been definitely seclusive if it had not been that he was put to school at 10 and left there until he was nearly 20, and so was forced to adapt himself to boyish life before the habit of retreating to the protection of his mother and family had become fixed. As he grew older he had a few abortive love affairs and became engaged the first year of the war. He is not yet married. As a child he had night terrors and a constant fear of the dark that clouded his childhood. As he grew older, however, he seems to have become much more normal, for he developed no phobias, had no nightmares, and none of the usual neurotic sensibilities, except for an undue horror of cruelty and bloodshed.

In the Spring of 1914 he had an attack of "neurasthenia" which he thinks was somewhat the same as his war neurosis. He was very much disappointed about the result of an examination which he had tried. When the telegram arrived announcing his failure he "sort of fainted," and was "hysterical" after that. For some weeks he slept poorly, had occasional nightmares, was easily fatigued, easily startled, and felt no ambition. This continued until the war broke out, shortly after which he joined the army and spent over a year in training for his artillery work. He rather enjoyed this, became quite sociable with his brother officers and looked forward keenly to going to France. He was rather curious to know what it would all be like. In his first shelling, no one was hit in his immediate vicinity. He became excited and enjoyed it in a sense. A few weeks later, when on a road back of the lines, a shell landed in the engine of a passing automobile and mangled the occupants horribly. This upset him a great deal and for a few weeks after the experience he stammered. (He gave a long and unnecessarily lurid account of this incident; in fact, in all his recitals there was evidence of a morbid fascination for him in the carnage of war.) Following this experience he always had some fear of shells, but as his battery was miles behind the front line trenches he was seldom under heavy or continuous bombardment.

After seeing what a shell could do, he always had a certain degree of abhorrence to the idea of killing people, but his victims were miles away and he kept from thinking of that aspect of his work too much, concentrating his mind rather on perfecting his technical skill in gunnery in which he was able to take considerable pride and satisfaction. He was quite sure that he never could be brought to the point of running a man through with a bayonet. He continued in this position for six weeks and then went home to England on leave. On returning, after being shelled again for the first time, he stammered for a day or two, but quickly recovered from this, and proceeded with his work comfortably enough for a good many months. He was then sent to Arras (in the Spring of 1917) and was there for nine weeks altogether. The fighting grew gradually heavier. He became tired with the constant strain, and began to be troubled with his fear of the shells. He became so nervous that he had to force himself to go through the communication trenches that were under shell fire. He slept less well, having difficulty in driving the thoughts of fighting from his mind, and had occasional dreams of running the battery, but no nightmares.

For the last four or five weeks the feeling grew that he could not keep on indefinitely and he began to wish that a shell would come and end it all. During this time he had great difficulty in putting from his mind thoughts of the wounds and death he was occasioning in the German lines. Finally, he was sent to an observation post in No-Man's-Land to direct the fire of one of his batteries. He went out a sap about fifty feet long that terminated under a pile of sand-bags through which there was a small loophole for observation. The Germans, evidently suspecting that an observer might be there, began to shell this spot pitilessly. The patient remained for some minutes with the shells bursting all around, and then retired to a dugout for about a quarter of an hour. Having recovered his courage, he returned to his post and made the necessary observations, although a great many shells were still falling. He thought that he might have received some slight concussion because his head ached a little, but otherwise he felt fairly comfortable. He was, however, very much strung up by his efforts, and a half hour later when he returned to his battery he fainted. The unconsciousness, if it was complete, lasted only a minute or so, but when he came to he was extremely fearful and so emotionally upset that he was sent back to a hospital at once. There he began to have the usual terrifying nightmares, in his case always of being shelled. On account of his poor sleep he was given sedatives very freely, the effect of which was to produce some sleep, it is true, but to make his nervous control very much less. As a result he got into a state where he was almost constantly shaking with violent, coarse tremors, and apt to show most dramatic exhibitions of fear when the slightest noise occurred. He stammered a good deal, but mainly when excited by examination, for he could speak quite calmly and consistently for several minutes without any hesitation. When under observation he frequently showed a peculiar tic. His lips would shut tight, with the corners of his mouth drawn back and up, his nose would be raised with a "pug" expression, both of which movements were coincident with a good deal of blinking and a slight retraction of the head. He seemed to be unaware of these contortions, but when they were described to him he said that those were the movements of his face and head when a shell burst and threw up earth near him, which seemed as if it would fly in his face. With this explanation, it was at once probable that the symptoms had developed from such actions of shrinking and disgust, for the expression of his face accurately showed these.

After six weeks in a general hospital, where he was subjected to a good deal of annoyance from the noises of busy wards and the sights of many wounded men, he was transferred to a special hospital in England. Here, under the influence of complete quiet and isolation, his symptoms very largely subsided in a matter of a couple of weeks. His dreams disappeared altogether, but he remained for a month, during which time I saw him occasionally, still prone to develop tremors, grimaces and signs of emotional instability when under close observation, or when startled by sudden noises. He was, however, anxious to understand the psychological mechanisms of his symptoms, and made promising efforts to gain complete control over himself.

CASE V. The following case gives an excellent example of the long fight which a patient may make against his symptoms, a struggle that reflects more credit on the individual than many exhibitions of sudden and unconscious courage. The patient is a lieutenant in the artillery, who joined the army in the Spring of 1915. He was always given to worrying about trifles, and to feeling that he had made mistakes. He was self-conscious, but with effort became steadily more sociable as he grew older. As a child he was painfully shy and fearful of his capacity to do anything. With adolescence he became more normal in this respect and had many puppy love affairs, and more serious ones, too, for he was finally married at the time he joined the army. Having seen little of his wife, he has had no change of outlook as the result of his marriage.

As a small boy he was afraid of the dark. He began reading when very young, and turned, boy-like, to books of adventure.

When night came, he would lie in the dark and people it with imaginations that would become very fearful. He has no memory, however, of actual nightmares. He has always been uncomfortable and disturbed during thunder-storms, although not exactly afraid. He invariably suffered from giddiness in high places, but has had no claustrophobic tendencies, and very few nightmares of any kind. Cruelty and bloodshed were always repulsive to him. As a boy, he played "Indian" a great deal with his brothers. The older brothers used to ambuscade him and scare him tremendously, even though he knew what was coming. His shyness kept him from playing team games as a boy, but when he was older he took up tennis, golf and walking, although music and reading were always his main interests. When he was 16, one of his brothers died of tuberculosis at the age of 23. A couple of years later, another brother died of the same disease at the same age. The patient became so obsessed by the fear that he himself would have tuberculosis that he was practically incapacitated and developed mild compulsive symptoms. When he passed the "danger period" at 23, however, he regained his confidence and shook off the fear of tuberculosis very largely.

He joined the army in the Spring of 1915 and remained in England under training for a year and a half. This was distinctly to his advantage, for he gained more confidence in himself and felt that he had become a competent individual. During this period he had no anxiety, and was philosophically resigned to whatever might happen in France. He went there in January, 1917, and was glad to find that conditions were better than he had been led to expect. When shelled for the first time he became worried rather than frightened, and quickly got used to it. It was possible for him to have shells drop quite close to him without being at all frightened. When he had been fighting for about six weeks he caught cold, had a bad tracheitis and bronchitis and lost his voice. When coughing, he brought up blood several times and of course began at once to worry about tuberculosis. With the natural physical strain of this infection, added to the worry, he felt very much dragged down and fatigued and continued so for about ten days. Then two 5·9 shells dropped, one ten, the other thirteen feet from him. The concussion did not cause him to lose consciousness, but he became so excited that he could not talk sensibly and was incoherent for an hour at least. He went to bed, but could sleep very little, and in the morning he found himself horribly afraid and trembling. With great effort he kept himself at work for a few days, and then was fortunate enough to be sent away for a course of study for twelve days. During this time he recovered from his fatigue, but worried constantly about having to return to his batteries and could not concentrate on his study. He went back to the line apprehensive of what might happen. The difficulty of continuing in his work became cumulatively greater. He was "jumpy" during the day, in constant fear of the shells, but keyed himself up to the task. At night he was always dreaming of being wounded in a ghastly fashion, and for some time had more fear of being wounded than of being killed. Before long, however, he reached the stage of wishing a shell would end his troubles completely and began to spend a good deal of time alone in planning some form of suicide that would afterward seem to have been an accident. For five or six weeks the struggle continued, although he felt more and more that it would be impossible for him to "carry on" indefinitely. About this time he was in the open one day and a German field gunner spied him and tried to hit him with twenty or thirty shells. This experience almost finished him, and he became so upset that his battery commander sent him to take charge of a wagon line in order that he might have less trying work. Although in less danger here, there were other worries from which he was not free. Always rather sensitive to the horrors of war, he now became obsessed by them, and marvelled continually that the whole ghastly business could be possible. He said later that he thought it was not improbable that he may have clenched his hands and shrieked at the horror of anything so cruel existing. When awake, this was his strongest feeling. Another symptom also developed. This was a difficulty in uttering guttural sounds, which soon spread to include all phonation, making him stammer constantly.

When it was later suggested to him that this may have been connected psychologically with the loss of his voice and fear of tuberculosis, he admitted that this was probably the case, inasmuch as these fears were much in his mind at the time the speech difficulty began.

In spite of these troubles he continued working for about a month longer, although the effort must have been great, considering that he had very little sleep, interrupted by nightmares, and that during the day he was both excessively fatigued and obsessed with horror. Altogether he had struggled on, in spite of these harrowing symptoms, for three and a half months! Finally, however, his superior officer sent him to divisional headquarters. There he got so much worse that he had to be sent almost immediately to a hospital. Once there, it seemed to him that if he were ever sent back to the line he would go mad. He was so depressed at the thought of his failure and the conviction that he was a coward that he frequently cried. The hospital he was in for nearly a month was next to a parade ground and at night they practised gunnery. With his extreme sensitiveness to sounds this terrorized him. Then he was removed to a hospital in London, where he improved quite rapidly, so that his main symptoms became not so much anxiety with its accompaniments as depression and an obsession with the wickedness and horror of war. This latter was developed to such a point that he was able to take absolutely no interest in such striking events as the capture of Messines Ridge which occurred while he was in the London hospital. He said that he was able to think of nothing but the carnage that must have taken place there. He felt, however, that this attitude was distinctly abnormal, in fact, that it was one of his difficulties. Wicked and horrible as war might be, he spontaneously admitted that in the present situation one's duty was not to think about it, but to fight, and end the struggle as soon as possible. At the same time he knew that it was his thinking about it which incapacitated him.

When he was first put in the hospital, the horrible sights at his last station were constantly before his eyes, as well as the immediate hospital surroundings. This lasted only a few days and then it became a matter not of seeing but merely of thinking about the bloodshed. Finally, he reached in London the point where he was able to drive these thoughts out of his mind by an effort of will, or where he could read a little and so distract his mind.

His dreams are of interest. In the latter part of his stay in the line, and for the first month in hospital, he dreamed constantly of working with his battery and being under shell fire, and this dream was consistently accompanied with great terror. When he began to recover, he had, with these previous stereotyped dreams, another recurring one. He was in the country near his home, which distantly resembled the country in France where his battery was. He was under shell fire, which he returned, but always with decreasing effect, so that his battery was gradually shelled out. In these dreams he would sometimes leave the battery and run, alone. At other times he would run with another officer. Occasionally the brigadier was with him, who looked on and criticized during the fighting. The brigadier, however, always disappeared before he had to run from the guns. The scenery of his home was not the only matter external to war that appeared in the setting of his dreams, for he began to replace his gunners with people he would read of during the day. Finally, dreams occurred that showed a direct regression to childhood, and the relation between the object of fear in his early life and what stimulated that emotion in the war. He began to dream, not that he was fighting against Germans, but that Indians were his foes.

This case is interesting both clinically and psychologically. We have an individual who showed strong neurotic tendencies before the war, who adapted himself only briefly to it, and then developed symptoms after his resistance was reduced by a worry that originated in times of peace. His dreams, too, showed a tendency to include material outside of war, and finally became a distortion of the great fear of his childhood, namely, that of Indians. He was constitutionally afflicted with a disgust of bloodshed and violence, and this became in his neurosis the most prominent factor in disabling him from active service. Running parallel to this were certain clinical features. The symptoms of pure and simple fatigue were less prominent in this case than is usual, and his disease was always much more subjective than objective. He had at any time very little nervous starting, and when I examined him, six weeks after his first admission to a hospital, he showed no tendency to jump when noises occurred, but was obviously greatly irritated by them. He had a little restlessness, and stammered pretty constantly in his speech, although the latter was steadily improving.

The next case, that of a lieutenant, aged 20, illustrates the effect of war on one who had always been considered rather below par nervously. Strictly speaking, this is not an anxiety case, in fact all the symptoms he showed were those which are usually merely complications in the anxiety neurosis. It is included here, however, as an example of the very much poorer adaptation made in war time by those who are not completely adapted to the demands of civil life, at the time they enter the army.

CASE VI. As a child he had frequent night terrors and was afraid of the dark. As he grew older he was high-strung and could not find himself at an elevation without wanting to throw himself down. He was never horrified by seeing animals killed but took a delight in it. He was shy with both sexes. He played games in moderation only, because he was never able to run any great distance. In fact, his father, who was a physician, took him from school at the age of 15 on account of his lack of strength, and discouraged him from the idea of studying medicine because he was too nervous. He was always subject to headaches which were somewhat improved by glasses.

In training his first symptom developed, which was a sharp pain in the left groin that got better when he lay down. This was apparently hysterical, as no physical reason could be found for it. After this he began to have shortness of breath, pain above the heart and palpitations, with occasional attacks of dizziness. He was absent on sick leave for a while. His superior officer did not wish him to go to the front, but he insisted on it, and was finally sent to France in September, 1916, after he had been seventeen months in training. He found himself at first somewhat afraid of the shells, but soon got used to them. The horror of the war, however, grew on him, and he came to pity the Germans as much as the British. His weakness, however, was his main difficulty, for he had to lie down half the time. This he regarded as failure and became depressed over it. Then his commanding officer committed suicide, and the idea of his doing this also obsessed him to such an extent that he thought he was going mad. He drove a knife into his upper lip and smashed a looking-glass because he hated to see himself. An extra long spell of duty in the trenches made him incapable of any further effort and he was sent home. In the hospital in England his chief difficulties were depression and thoughts of suicide and a desire to mutilate himself. As to the latter, he at first feared that he would do himself serious harm; but later he discovered that a slight pain and the drawing of blood gave him the satisfaction he seemed to crave. His chief trouble was the lack of any confidence in himself. His failure, as such, ceased to bother him, and he rationalized that comfortably with the conviction that he should never have been sent to the front. He complained, too, of lack of memory and concentration. His reaction was typically neurotic and offered more difficulty in the way of treatment than the usual war neurosis. He insisted that he was physically incapable of outdoor exercise, yet always complained of a headache if he stayed indoors. He said he wanted to go back to the front, but he knew that he couldn't, and refused to consider the possibility of getting well with the idea of doing some work at home. Therefore, he argued, there was nothing left for him but to think of suicide.

As he showed no signs of organic heart trouble physically, one is safe in assuming that these symptoms were largely, if not entirely, neurotic, and that the patient was an individual not quite capable of meeting the ordinary strain and stress of civil life, consequently far from competent to deal with the strain of war.

The following case is also not typical, but is included here to show how what is essentially a peace neurosis may develop symptoms that are coloured by the environment of war.

CASE VII.  The patient is a captain in the French Army, attached as a liaison officer to the British staff.  At the time I saw him he had returned to duty and was good enough to give me a retrospective account of his neurosis.

He had a severe attack of meningitis at 3, and as a result, was very delicate as a child.  It was not thought by his parents that he ever would be strong enough to be educated, and he was given no schooling until he had himself demonstrated his intellectual ability.  He was always "nervous" but never had any definite symptoms and no breakdowns.  He became a barrister and passed successfully many examinations both in France and in England.  It is important to note that he had very little anxiety in connexion with any of his examinations.  He was commissioned immediately at the outbreak of the war, and fought for some months with the French Army.  Shortly after the beginning of the war he got news of the death of his best friend.  At once he began having dreams of examinations, in which failure seemed certain, and was tormented by great fear of this.  There were other dreams of his arguing in court most ineffectively, in fact so poorly that his clients insulted him.  He was tired in the morning after these dreams.  Under this strain he soon began to be nervous and fearful of shells, but never showed this fear, and in fact felt it less, when he was in the company of others.  He had no increase of horror at the carnage, but could never become accustomed to shell fire.  After continuing in this state for eighteen months, and, so far as he could remember, without any particular aggravation of his difficulties, he fell in a "fit" while drilling some men.  He was told that he did not have a convulsion, but talked as if he were apologizing to the colonel.  Following this, he was extremely weak and had bad pains in his legs; when he walked it was with a very staggering gait and exaggerated movements.  He was, of course, incapable of fighting further, and was sent to the south of France.  He stayed there very quietly with his wife for nearly five months, for the first two of which he felt absolutely no affection for his wife.  All this time he endeavoured to rest completely, and did not even read a newspaper.  This was apparently successful treatment, for he recovered completely, and on returning to the front felt no more fear and had perfect confidence in himself. Later he obtained leave long enough to go to London for some English bar examinations, which he passed without having any anxiety at all. He continued, however, to repress his friend's death, trying never to think about it, and was always disturbed for some time after hearing the friend's name mentioned.

# CHAPTER V

## FATIGUE

PERHAPS the most important of all the factors that unite in the production of an anxiety state is fatigue. So far as I have been able to learn, either it or concussion is present to greater or less extent in every case of anxiety neurosis, and it seems to be possible to trace its influence directly in the production of symptoms.

Although the discrimination may be somewhat academic, it is possible to recognize two types of fatigue which are usually combined. These we might call physical and mental in origin, although there is probably no place in medicine where it is more difficult to discriminate between what is purely physical and purely mental. We may call fatigue physical in origin that proceeds from physical factors outside the patient, such as continued exertion on duty, exposure to inclement weather, lack of food and opportunity to sleep, or physical disease. Fatigue of mental origin is that which proceeds from difficulties that are more psychological than physical in their operation. This includes the constant stress of exposure to what is extremely distasteful, whether the distaste be common to all mankind, or an idiosyncrasy of the patient. It also includes the fatigue coming from the struggle against symptoms already in existence. These influences rarely demand in times of peace the consideration due them in warfare. The reason for this is that escape from symptoms or from environmental factors which are particularly trying is usually possible to some extent in civil life, but is absolutely impossible in the trenches.

Two cases of the physical type may first be quoted:

CASE VIII. The patient is a lieutenant, aged 29, who was a regular soldier for eight years before the present war. He had an extraordinarily normal mental make-up, liked military life extremely, and did well in it, so that he was made a non-commissioned officer almost immediately after enlistment.　He went to France as a sergeant with the original expeditionary force, and went through all the severe fighting in the retreat from Mons and the first battle of Ypres, unscathed.

He exhibited no symptoms whatever with his first shell fire, and enjoyed the fighting hugely.　At the first, he did not like to "mess the dead about," but soon became quite indifferent to this part of his duties.　He was several times rather saddened by losing all his chums, but he was never unable to continue in his duties, and soon forgot about these incidents.　From the standpoint of adaptation he might easily be called a perfect soldier, for he was not only completely devoid of fear, but well disciplined, and took a keen enjoyment in his work and was able to continue fighting quite unaffected by the horrors that are trying to all ordinary individuals.　In August, 1915, he had a slight touch of rheumatism, not severe enough to send him to the hospital, but enough to drag him down a bit.　He thought that he had recovered completely from this.　Two or three months later the Germans exploded a mine right in front of the trench in which he was.　This is perhaps quite the most fearful event in any soldier's life, as all the ground is shaken and the extent of the damage done may be appalling.　The patient went pale for the first time in his life, but did not lose his control, and kept his men "standing to" immediately.　It was a new experience to him and rather a shock.　He began to think for the first time about danger.　He was in an area where mining was the chief form of attack, and he would frequently hear the Germans digging beneath his dugout.　He got too restless to sleep while on active duty, but could sleep well when back in billets.　This continued for two months, during which time, he thinks now, he was probably getting worse than he realized at the time.　He was getting more and more on edge, although he felt no real fear, and could always tell by the sounds where shells were going to land.　About six weeks after the mining incident, he was buried in a dugout.　He did not completely lose consciousness, but was so dazed that he had to lie down for a couple of hours. Following this, he was nervous, had a chronic headache and could not sleep, even in the billets. He would lie for a long time, trying to get to sleep, his head aching, seeing dugouts being blown out, and the men being bowled over, and imagining himself in the way of shells. Occasionally he could feel these things as well as see them, but could always by an effort of will convince himself that they were only imaginations. With these hallucinations he had no real fear, but was very much bothered and wished they would go away. All this time he was in a position of the most trying responsibility which any non-commissioned officer can have, since he was company sergeant-major. Feeling this responsibility, he continued his work, but got gradually worse and worse. His sleep became poorer. Not that he had nightmares, but he found himself constantly awaking with a start whenever he fell off to sleep. In the daytime he was bothered by a constant tendency to "jump" whenever a shell came, but was able to keep himself perfectly calm as far as any outsider could see. It was only with the greatest effort, however, that he was able to get through each day. He began taking morphia, but was able to secure very little sleep with it. He thought sometimes of suicide.

After two months of these troublesome symptoms, his officers saw that he was not well and sent him to England. Here he picked up quickly. He soon began to sleep a little, but he never was able to get more than five hours' sleep in any night. After a rest of three months he applied for some light duty, and was given company accountant work. This soon bored him extremely, and, as he insisted on returning to France, he was given a commission and sent back to the front in January, 1917, after he had been nine months in England. On his return, he found the fighting not very active, and was able to go ahead with it very well for a while, with his condition about the same as in England; that is, he felt rather high-strung and was able to get only four or five hours' sleep at night. In April he was sent to Arras. A month before this he had a dream that he was going to be bowled over by a shell, buried, and wounded in the neck.

4—2

He thought a good deal about this, and realized perfectly that he was not thoroughly fit. At Arras, where the fighting was very heavy, his sleep got much poorer. He had, however, no "jumpiness," nor any idea of suicide. Then in April he led his men in an advance, and almost immediately on leaving the trench was bowled over and buried by a shell and at the same time hit in the neck, knee, and the hand (all superficial wounds). He was not unconscious, but dazed and had to be carried back to the hospital. There he felt first rather pounded and blinded, but slept a little, and was fairly comfortable after ten days. In fact, he felt so much better that he undertook a journey down to his base. This exhausted him and he arrived almost in a collapse. He was in camp at the base for three weeks, during which time he tried to rest, and took tonics, but got steadily worse. He became depressed, thinking that something was going to happen and kill him. It was not exactly a shell, and he could not tell what it was to be,—it was just a restless, vague anxiety. He found that he could not concentrate his thoughts sufficiently to read. Occasionally he contemplated committing suicide in order to finish up quickly what was going to happen anyway. He had practically no sleep, but whenever he would doze, would wake with a start, feeling that something had hit him.

This was as near as he came to a real nightmare. He had several dreams of being taken prisoner. This probably expressed an unconscious relief from having to fight, but how far this was from his conscious ideals may be gathered from what took place on waking. He would immediately imagine himself in the situation of prisoner, and then in fancy start a fight and escape back to the British lines.

He was in various hospitals for two weeks, and then was sent to a special hospital for nervous cases which was very pleasantly situated in the country. Ten days in this quiet situation improved his condition considerably and he began to get some sleep. On a day after no sleep, he would have a bad headache, be restless and apprehensive, with a feeling that he would never get better, always being worse when he was alone. The distraction of talking to others did him good. Any exertion, however, would lead to a very bad headache. He thought that if he were left permanently alone he would go mad. At no time had he had real nightmares. It was quite interesting that he discovered when riding on a train that he would become terrorized on passing through every tunnel lest he should be crushed.

This case shows how incapacitating pure fatigue without the development of any marked neurotic symptoms may be. Judging from what one gathers in taking the histories of many patients, it might be safe to say that had this lieutenant's superiors not sent him back to the hospital after his final burial, he would have developed a typical anxiety state, for all the symptoms were potentially present. We can probably account for his long and successful struggle against a neurosis by the fact that he was so extraordinarily well adapted to fighting. But, as he himself said, "There is no man on earth who can stick this thing for ever."

The following case is interesting and typical in two respects. In the first place, he was a man well adapted to fighting, whose first symptoms were those of fatigue, apart from any neurotic manifestations. Secondly, his neurosis, once established, remained in abeyance for thirteen months while at home only to blossom out immediately on his return to the front.

CASE IX. The patient is a lieutenant, aged 21, who showed no distinctly neurotic tendencies. He was somewhat shy with girls and slightly so with boys, but played many games with them, and seems to have been rather a normal child. His only abnormality, apparently, was a tendency to self-consciousness. He enlisted in September, 1914, and found that the training did him much good, for he became more sociable; it "made a man of him," as he said. He went to France in February, 1915, and although he was at first somewhat frightened, soon got used to being shelled. He enjoyed the life and was careless of the sight of wounds and death.

After fighting for seven months, he became somewhat fatigued and had occasional dreams of fighting, with fear. In the daytime, however, he had only a tendency to start when the shells came, and no consciousness of fear whatever. He was then

invalided home with a fever, and three months later was given
a commission, spending nine months in training.  He then returned to France as an officer in October, 1916.  He at once
joined a company which had just been in severe action and was
feeling very shaky.  This had some effect on him, and he found
himself slightly nervous and a little depressed at the thought of
going back to the firing line.  He tried to persuade himself that
he did not care what happened.  When examined later, he told
me that this initial fear was probably due to the rough time he
had before he left the firing line thirteen months earlier.  He had
never, in all the time he was at home, gained complete possession
of his confidence.  He found now that he could get no enjoyment
in the fighting, and became sensitive to the horrors.  He began
to take rum in order to keep fit.  The fighting was so active that
he had little opportunity to sleep, but when he did have the
chance he was not bothered by bad dreams.  Gradually he became more and more frightened, but was constantly successful
in hiding any signs of it.  The fatigue became so extreme that he
felt that it could not last long, and wished fervently that a shell
would come along and finish him.

One night a raid was on, and a heavy barrage.  He remembered
nothing more until he awoke in a dressing station where he was
told that he had been buried.  Apparently he had been unconscious for three or four hours.  His head ached, as did his back,
where the earth had hit it.  He had no dizziness, no further loss
of consciousness and no difficulty in thinking.  As there is no
evidence of concussion, except from his amnesia, it is probable
that it was rather slight.  He felt very much frightened, however,
but managed to get some control of this as he was carried further
from the firing line back to the field ambulance.  He remained
here ten days, and recovered sufficiently to insist on being sent
back.  He found on his return to the line, however, that he could
not sleep, and was extremely frightened during the day.  He
realized at once that he could not stick it out, and after a week
asked to be sent back.  This was done at once, and he was sent
direct to England.  He was in the hospital for a week where his
sleep was very poor and continuously troubled by nightmares,

the content of which was exclusively a repetition of previous terrifying incidents at the front. He was extremely shaky; in fact, his legs moved so much that he crossed them in bed in order to keep them quiet. This extreme shakiness he ascribed not only to his nervous strain, but also to the injury to his back, which remained sore for some time, and which he thought included an injury to his spinal cord which was responsible for the movements of his legs. At the end of the week he got up out of bed in order to return to his home. He then found that he could not uncross his legs, and was so spastic that he had great difficulty in walking. In his home, his family and friends exhausted him by their constant efforts to distract his mind. He was very restless, and his dreams became more insistent at night. He remained at home three and a half months, during which time his fatigue, shakiness, sleeplessness, all appeared worse. His dreams, however, became less severe, in that they appeared at less frequent intervals. He was then sent to a special hospital where I saw him after two months' stay. He had improved in all directions. The dreams had ceased. He had no chronic fatigue, although he was still rather easily fatigable. The shakiness had disappeared except when he was tired or when he tried to stand or walk with his legs apart. His gait, however, was improving very rapidly under the methods of re-education which were employed.

He said that he kept himself from thinking much about returning to France, but when that idea did come in his mind it was always accompanied with a fear that he would be a coward if he were once back in the firing line again. He worried a good deal about his failure, because he had seen a good deal of prejudice against a man who "goes sick," whatever the cause.

It may probably be taken as additional evidence of this patient's essential normality, that he had no trouble whatever in abstaining from alcohol after leaving the line, although he had been afraid that he would have difficulty in this.

The following two cases are illustrative of fatigue engendered by mental as well as physical difficulties, and difficulties, too, that would not be at all incapacitating in times of peace with as normal individuals as these patients are.

CASE X. The patient is a major, aged 35, who had spent seven
years in the army with the rank of captain, but had resigned
some five years previous to the beginning of the present war.
During this time he had been living in North Africa, engaged for
some years in tribal warfare, and following that had built a
plantation miles from civilization where he lived very happily.
He is a typical representative of the British adventuring, colon-
izing class.  At the beginning of the war he returned to England
and was given a commission as major, and fought for two years
before his breakdown occurred.  In make-up he was apparently
an unusually normal individual, and in many talks with him I
could discover no abnormality except that he was a confirmed
bachelor, and that he was always unusually antagonistic to inefficiency in any superior.

On going to France, after a short initial period of fear with the
shells, he became fully adapted to the conditions and enjoyed
the fighting.  Probably as a result of his many years of life in
the open, he knew how to adapt himself to an uncivilized environment, and took considerable pride in making not only himself, but all his men, unusually comfortable.  He fought continuously for one and one-half years, with absolutely no symptoms.  At one time, when he was feeling particularly fit, he was
in a dugout with two other men when a heavy, high explosive
shell pierced the roof and exploded.  All three men were laid out
immediately, and all apparently paralyzed for half an hour.
The patient said he thought he might have been unconscious
for a second or two.  It was difficult to recall his sensations.  He
remembered being very much frightened, but what occasioned
that fear he cannot remember.  He also was unable to say
whether he was really paralyzed or unable to move, or perhaps
afraid to move.  At any rate, at the end of the half hour all three
men picked themselves up, laughed at each other and went on
with their work.  The patient felt no after-effects whatever.  As
such an incident is frequently given as the occasion of a neurosis,
it is important to note how little effect it may have on those who
have not been troubled with any symptoms prior to the event.

After a year and a half of fighting, the patient was transferred to a battalion that was under the command of a brigadier whom he felt to be not only very inefficient, but antagonistic to him. They had frequent difference on various matters, and finally when they disagreed on tactics, the brigadier had him sent home on sick leave, although he was perfectly well. He returned to the front after a few months' stay at home, and was very much disappointed to be transferred to the same division and come under the authority of his old enemy ten months after leaving him.

Up to this time he felt perfectly well, but the strain of constantly following orders of which he did not approve, began to tell on him. He became sleepless at night, and "jumpy" during the day. This "jumpiness" at first was not accompanied by fear, but later on he became fearful of the shells. Much irritated by this failure, he made strong efforts to control his emotion, and did succeed in hiding it from his brother officers and from his men. The brigadier, however, continued to bother him in every possible way, so the patient thought. He was continually pestered for reports, so that he had to spend much time in purely clerical work. He began to dream of this. Night after night he would be making endless inventories which he never was able to finish, so that he would wake in the morning more tired than when he had gone to sleep. Finally the patient and his brigadier came to an open quarrel about a case of court martial when the patient accused his superior of attempting to coerce the court illegally. The brigadier over-ruled him, but was possibly in the wrong as he made no complaint of the patient's actions to headquarters. As the patient had begun to have occasional terrifying dreams of fighting at night, he felt that his resistance was steadily decreasing. He tried taking bromides in ten grain doses every night for some weeks, but finally discontinued the use of this drug because he found it was failing to give any benefit at this dosage. He had been on active service for many months, so felt justified in applying for leave. This was granted and he came to London. There he consulted a neurologist who advised him to go to a hospital, which he did at once. He showed some tremulousness, but no other obvious abnormality, and his subjective symptoms were not so intense as is often the case. His nightmares occurred regularly every night, only for about a week, after which they became fewer in number, and after two weeks disappeared entirely. Sleeplessness, however, continued to bother him, and sometimes he would lie awake practically the whole night rehearsing in his mind the past quarrels with the brigadier, or imaginary defiances.

After two or three weeks' stay in the hospital he began to go out for occasional walks or rides in a motor, and he was then disgusted to find how easily he was fatigued and how fearful he was of the traffic. After a month of hospital residence he went to a convalescent home in the country, from which he wrote me a month later to state that, although he had no obvious symptoms, his convalescence was proceeding much more slowly than he had expected. He found himself still nervous with any sudden noise, terribly giddy if he were in a high place, and much upset by thunder-storms. In addition, he could not entirely shake himself of the obsession concerning the brigadier. Unfortunately there was no opportunity for any psychological analysis of this antagonism to his superior, but judging from the experience of others with such cases, it seems probable that it would have been a comparatively simple matter to give this patient insight into and control over his trouble.

It is probably safe to say in this case that the main factor in the patient's breakdown was his constitutional inability to act subserviently and take orders from one whom he did not respect. This spirit is, of course, an asset in times of peace. In military life, however, it is a distinct disadvantage.

CASE XI. The history of this patient presents a somewhat similar situation to that just described. He was commissioned in the regular army in 1906, became an officer in the artillery, and enjoyed the army life. When the war broke out he was home on sick leave from India and joined the expeditionary force in France in November, 1914. His make-up showed that he had not been a completely normal individual. As a child he had many nightmares of falling and was also afraid of the dark. This latter fear never entirely left him, for he stated to me that he thought he probably would be still afraid to remain alone in a dark house. He showed no other obviously neurotic tendencies, but admitted himself to be given to worry, and to being over-conscientious. He confessed to a distinct vein of pessimism. He had, too, a strong tendency to be unusually resentful when deceived or ill-treated. As an example, he spoke of once being decoyed into buying some trash at an auction sale. After discovering the worthlessness of the things he thought and dreamed about the deceit that had been practised on him for some months. He felt very resentful at the auctioneer and indulged in phantasies of revenge. Both his father and grandfather had been soldiers of some eminence, and the ideals of military service took a large place in his life. After being commissioned he had frequent dreams of being in the army without having passed the necessary examinations. In these dreams he felt that these examinations were still to come, and that he was going to fail. On waking, this feeling would persist for some time, with considerable depression.

On going to France he fought continuously for many months and enjoyed it. When first shelled he wanted to leave, but had no other abnormal reactions. Occasionally he would feel a little timorous when going into the front line trenches for observation of the effect of his battery's work. This feeling was always quite brief, however, and never incapacitated him. After eight months of fighting he was one day very heavily shelled, after which he was "jumpy" and for some weeks every sound he heard meant a shell. He recovered from this spontaneously, however.

From May to November, 1916, he acted as liaison artillery officer with the flying corps. He enjoyed this work extremely and felt so full of life that, although it was not at all a part of his duties, he used to go on bombing raids for the fun of it. He did not enjoy being shot at by the anti-aircraft guns, but was never sufficiently frightened to develop any symptoms whatever. After five months of this work, he felt that he was not doing all that he might, and so applied for a position in the artillery again. He was sent home to raise and train a new siege battery. His troubles then began. None of his officers or men had ever been in France, so that he had to instruct all of them in many essentials. An additional difficulty was that he was forced by regulations to teach methods which he had not seen in use at the front, and which he thought the men would only have to forget again. At the end of this period he spent two weeks giving the battery firing-practice which he thought ought to have been extended to six months. He worried morbidly about the insufficiency of training which his men were getting, and felt that he was up against a system more powerful than himself. To add to his difficulties he had innumerable administrative duties to attend to that he found very irksome.

A week before going to France he had a bad throat. His physician kept him in bed for two days, and said that his rest ought to be continued for a month as he was worn out and his heart was irregular in action. He left his bed, however, to go over to France, feeling quite played out. He spent ten days tuning up his tractors, etc., and then to his intense disappointment his guns were taken from him, as they were urgently needed for another sector of the line than that to which he had been ordered. He and his men were sent to build gun positions for another offensive that was to take place months later. Difficulties began once again. He had not, or felt that he had not, enough men, material or transport facilities. Finally, the general over-ruled his judgment as to where the emplacements should be. The patient felt that a terrible mistake was being made, and it became an obsession to him. On going to sleep at night it was in his mind, and although he did not dream of it, he never slept more than four hours and found himself thinking at once of the same subject when he awoke. While continuing in his work, he saw a neighbouring battery knocked out by German shells, and began to live over in prospect the experiences the batteries he was building would have in the future.

Next, the Germans began to shell all the roads back of the British lines, indiscriminately, which drove his men into a panic. He managed to put some confidence in them again, but only with great difficulty, and he himself was beginning to wish urgently that a shell might hit him, so that he might get a wound which would remove him from duty. It is interesting that he did not wish for death—the only officer I examined who did not look for this form of release. It was probably because he felt so outraged with the "system" that he harboured the less honourable wish. On the other hand, when his doctor recommended a ten days' rest, the patient refused, being stubbornly determined to stick it out. He was given thirty grains of bromide a day which improved his condition, but only for a few days. He had been working under these difficulties for six weeks when he was given orders that he considered impossible of completion in the time allowed. This made matters even worse and he got so that he could not eat, nor concentrate his mind sufficiently even for the purpose of reading orders. He was also trembling most of the time, and starting nervously whenever shells came, although he felt no fear of them, in fact they had a definite, conscious attraction for him. Finally, he saw several men injured and one killed working on a gun emplacement the location of which he had protested against. The following day he was ordered to undo all his work and remove the emplacement to another spot. This was more than he could bear, so he went to the doctor again and demanded relief from all responsibility. He was sent to a hospital, and had been in one hospital or another for six weeks when I saw him.

He experienced great relief in leaving the line, but still had other difficulties indicative of fatigue. He was "jumpy" and felt that he was gripping hard on things in order to keep control of himself. He spoke in a fixed tone and felt he was mentally incompetent. Paraldehyde gave him sleep for one night, but left him heavy for several days following. When the sleeplessness passed, he was still weak. He was in bed for ten days altogether. Then he dreamed several nights in succession of working on his gun emplacements. This upset him once more, but only temporarily. His sleep finally became quite normal, but he continued to suffer with headaches and difficulty in concentration. His greatest difficulty when I saw him was depression with a feeling of failure. He feared that having broken down in a crisis, his future career as a soldier would be prejudiced. He continued to harbour resentment against the superiors from whom he had suffered, but spontaneously developed more and more insight into the fact that his own reaction had not been perfectly normal.

This case presents some interesting points for speculation. The origin of his fatigue is plain enough, but we have to account for so marked a degree of fatigue not culminating in an anxiety condition. Two possibilities must be considered. In the first place, he never desired death as a release from his situation, which seems to be a pretty constant forerunner of the anxiety state. Secondly, his mental conflict remained quite conscious throughout. It is possible that there was in his case less necessity for the development of neurotic symptoms in that he had an open, conscious antagonism to the military situation in which he was placed.

# CHAPTER VI

## CONCUSSION

THE role of concussion in the production of anxiety states has been emphasized by the more organically minded neurologists with probably too great an emphasis. On the other hand, those who have been working psychologically seem inclined to under-estimate its importance, and, so far as I know, neither school has attempted to make any discrimination, in their reported cases, between the symptoms which could be directly accounted for on this physical basis, and those which were more probably purely psychological in origin. In less than a fourth of the cases I have seen could concussion be determined as a preponderating factor. Two-thirds had no suggestion whatever of concussion in their history. That it is rarely, if ever, the sole factor is suggested by the phenomena not infrequently reported, that many men are often equally affected by the same explosion, while only some of them develop symptoms. It has also been stated that cases have occurred where a shell has dropped among a group of men who were resting. One who was awake developed "shell shock." Those who were asleep showed no bad effects. Perhaps the most convincing argument of all is that the same man may be repeatedly exposed to definite concussion at times when his general condition is perfect, and develop only the most tem-porary symptoms, whereas later in his career as a soldier when fatigue or beginning neurotic symptoms are present, a less violent concussion may precipitate a severe neurosis.

By examining cases with definite history of severe concussion one can discover the symptoms which are the direct outcome of the physical injury. These are as follows:

There is first unconsciousness that may last for hours, even days. Lumbar puncture at this time may, according to the reports, show blood in the cerebro-spinal fluid. That there are minute hemorrhages throughout the brain has been determined definitely in some cases which have been killed instantly by concussion, and it is also suggested by the fact that retinal hemorrhages may frequently be observed ophthalmoscopically. When consciousness is recovered it does not remain immediately and permanently clear, as the patient is apt to go through a period of hours or days in which he is constantly drifting off into unconsciousness or sleep. Sometimes consciousness may be retained for a longer period, when the patient's attention is continuously stimulated. Retention of urine or incontinence of both urine and faeces is common in these stages. Many of the patients, on becoming clear, are aphasic. A period of delirium then is apt to ensue, during which the patient imagines himself to be fighting again. This delirium is distinctly of the occupational type, and so far as I could learn, is not accompanied by fear unless neurotic symptoms had been present before the concussion, or the patient has an extremely abnormal make-up. The patient may gain insight into the unreality of his hallucinations if his attention is forcibly directed to his environment. In fact, the delirium is apt to disappear slowly as the patient gets to do this more and more for himself. He is then in a condition of great fatigue and extremely poor mental tension, the last being demonstrated by a difficulty in collecting his thoughts, defective orientation, poor memory for the remote past, and practically no memory at all for the immediate past. Generally there is retroactive amnesia for the concussion itself, and for a varying lapse of time prior to the accident. All mental operations are performed with great difficulty, and as a rule inaccurately, which can easily be tested by demanding some simple calculations. The voice is peculiar, being very often pitched somewhat higher than is usual for the patient, monotonous, and frequently slow, words being separated by a pause of one or two seconds. The patient begins with greater or less speed, according to the severity of his injury, to recover his memory of the remote past, and also, strangely enough, is frequently able to reconstruct a good deal of the period which immediately preceded his injury, particularly if some hints are given him. In the milder cases the patient feels as well as he ever did, after a few weeks' rest.

In the more severe cases, some symptoms are apt to persist. For a long time the patient has poor mental tension, and this is so frequently associated with carelessness and with the brief appearance of fanciful ideas, that a.suspicion of paresis is often aroused. Occasionally the patient may retain delusions for months that originated in his initial delirium.

The importance of knowing these symptoms lies in the fact that their presence in the clinical history (particularly the dipping of consciousness and poor mental tension) is a tell-tale sign of genuine concussion. They are singularly absent in the cases where mere burial, or some other such precipitating cause, has suddenly produced symptoms. In those individuals where definite fatigue or neurotic symptoms are already present, even in slight degree, the occurrence of concussion may cause a very sudden accentuation in the anxiety picture. The following two cases illustrate the effects of concussion on individuals previously normal in their make-up and in good health when the accident occurred:

CASE XII. The patient is a Canadian from Toronto, aged 20. His personal history shows an extremely normal make-up. In 1915 he lost the phalanges and metatarsals of his left foot in a railway accident. This injury prevented his acceptance by the Canadian military authorities for a long time, but finally he was commissioned in the English Royal Flying Corps. He spent nine months in England in training, which he enjoyed greatly, and at the end of that time he was considered sufficiently competent to be sent to France. He made several successful flights over the lines, but after only two weeks of service he was shot down and crashed to the ground within his own lines. He was removed at once to a British general hospital, where twenty-four hours later he was noted as being still unconscious, with black eyes and bruises on his body, but no neurological signs. Four days later he had apparently recovered consciousness, and had complete control of his sphincters. A week later, it is stated that his memory was much aided by questions, but that he was still hazy about recent events. He could recognize that he was in the hospital, but was not sure which one it was. A week after this again, he arrived in a London hospital[1]. Here he refused to stay in bed and was found, by his physician, lying half covered, with bright eyes, and speaking in a very loud voice. Several questions were addressed to him, during which time he made no response, merely staring at his examiner as he moved around the bed. Finally, the patient shouted: "I want to get up." He was told he could not do so immediately, and then when questioned as to his orientation, he said that he was in Rosedale (a suburb of Toronto). Asked where Rosedale was, he insisted it was a part of London, that it was not far, that he wanted a taxicab to get there. When his physician told him that he would have to cross the ocean in order to get to Rosedale, he stared, but seemed content. His physician discovered a wound on his right hip (it looked like a superficial machine-gun wound). He asked the patient about it, who said he didn't know, but thought it must be the mark of a hospital he had been in in France. He expected the physician to know what it was, that it was a secret mark meaning that he could return to the line and fight whenever he wanted to. He also explained it as a mark indicating that he could use the lavatory whenever he wanted to.

He gave no answers to several questions as to personal data, and then suddenly exclaimed: "I want to go to Rosedale," but was easily quieted. When asked if he dreamed, he looked up with a cunning expression, and then said: "I down the Boche," —"I am a live wire,"—"he never lives,"—"I kill him." He was asked "Every time?" to which he replied: "I *kill* every time." During the utterance of these few phrases he became very excited.

The next day he was tractable, but anxious to leave and still asking about Rosedale. He wanted to leave at once. When asked where he was, he laughed, and said the nurse told him he was a long way from Rosedale, and when questioned as to his

[1] I am indebted to Captain Maurice Nicoll, R.A.M.C., for the use of his notes on the observations made in this hospital.

belief in this, said: "I guess I have to go in a train and in a ship," but seemed uncertain. Further conversation showed that he had assimilated considerable information gained from the nurses, and that he was much more thoroughly in touch with his environment. I saw him for a few minutes and told him I would see him again the following day in another hospital to which he was to be transferred. The next morning I found him oriented for time and able to recognize me with difficulty. He was much confused about the names of the hospitals, and his recent movements. None of the necessary data seemed ever to be absent from his mind, but to be present in rather a jumble. He showed a definite mental tension defect. He was not aware of being slowed in his mental processes, but admitted difficulty in recalling some data. In subtracting seven from one hundred serially, he did it very slowly, and made several bad mistakes, which he did not recognize. In giving an account of the remote past, he had difficulty in getting his facts straight, particularly in their right relations to one another. There were a number of discrepancies into which he had only partial insight. His carelessness concerning his intellectual defect was very striking, reminding one of the similar reaction in a paretic. He could recall no dreams at all, but remembered his life in France well enough to be sure that he had no nervous symptoms. He could give no account of any hypnagogic hallucinations. Although he was well enough oriented concerning his situation in England, the idea of getting to Canada was still in his mind, but he remarked a number of times that he must speak to the head of the hospital about it. Physically he admitted some fatigability, and complained of his eyesight, that things got foggy if he looked at them long. Nystagmus was present on looking to the extreme left. His optic disks showed haziness and redness with the margins obscured. The remains of one hemorrhage were seen.

Two weeks later he complained of waking early in the morning, but not of any other difficulties in sleeping. He said his memory was much better. He could remember my name and the name of the hospital where he had first seen me, and external events that had occurred on the day of my previous visit. He also said that memory of his last day of fighting was coming back. He could recall being chased by a German aeroplane, and thinking that his observer had shot the German down. He could also recall going through various manoeuvres in order to escape the German, and said that he suspected his aeroplane had been hit by an anti-aircraft gun.

He was still worried about going to Canada, this obsession now having taken the form of fearing that a medical board would send him directly back to France, that the board would not realize that he was incompetent to fly again, whereas he knew that he could not, because he had difficulty in telling "up" from "down," and was subject to some dizziness. He also felt that there was something the matter with his vision as things did not look perfectly clear to him. When tested, however, he seemed to have no defect. The nystagmus on looking to the left was still present and his left pupil was slightly larger than the right.

As the foregoing account shows, the patient developed no neurotic symptoms whatever, following this concussion, his difficulties being strictly of the organic type. There was first great confusion and disorientation, with some delirium-like ideas; following this, considerable recovery, as evidenced by grosser intellectual tests, but a persisting defect for grasping more subtle situations.

The next case gives an illustration of a less severe concussion, also without any neurotic reaction. The dreams he developed are of particular interest inasmuch as their content and the accompanying affect were distinctly different from those of the anxiety state:

CASE XIII. The patient is a major in the artillery, aged 39. He fought during the South African war and had been in the regular army all his adult life. There was no trace of abnormality. to be discovered in his make-up, in fact, he had an extremely open, pleasant personality. He fought until the end of May, 1917, without ever developing real symptoms. He was wounded three times, though none of the wounds were serious. Once after being wounded he had a few nightmares, but could not recall the content of them.

At the beginning of March he was sent with his battery to the Messines region and was extremely busy preparing for and assisting in the final bombardment. On June 3, after having worked very hard, he was tired and lay down in his dugout to rest. Although feeling weary, he had developed no symptoms indicative of real fatigue and had had no bad dreams or "jumpiness." He remembers that the battery was being bombarded and that he heard two 5·9 shells land near the battery. The last he remembers was reading some dispatches and turning them over to his captain. His next memory was of awakening in a casualty clearing station. A shell had pierced the roof of his dugout, had killed three and wounded nine, and broken up the bed on which he was lying. Some iron from the bedstead hit him in the abdomen. The shell fire was so heavy that those in the dugout could not be rescued for some time. Then the patient was dragged out into a field. He was partly conscious, but fainted in the field. When he recovered from this he insisted on going to the battery and taking charge of it. His junior officers saw that he was quite dazed and hopelessly incompetent, but were unable to get him to leave his post until they told him that the brigadier had ordered him to headquarters. He went to headquarters and there became confused again, so that he was removed to the casualty clearing station. His memories began three or four days after the concussion. The first memory was of this hospital being under shell fire, which did not frighten him. For about a week he had intense pain in his abdomen, particularly on micturition, but that soon left him entirely. His head ached and he had a big bruise on the occiput, and he suffered from intense photophobia and poor vision. There was considerable difficulty in talking as he found it hard to get the right words. After a week in this hospital he was transferred to London. There he was slightly confused and disoriented and troubled by his dreams which recurred every night and disturbed his sleep. I saw him a couple of days after this when his confusion had cleared up, objectively at least. He spoke in a monotonous slow voice with pauses between the phrases as if it were an effort to talk, and it seemed as if he had occasional difficulty in finding the right word. The pitch of his voice was unnaturally high and had a distinct monotony that was in marked contrast to his emotional normality. In spite of the distress he was in, he talked fully and pleasantly about his experiences. His chief complaints were of pain in the head, weakness and "shakiness." This last was not objectively visible, but probably was his term to describe his fatigue. He was unable to give any clear account of events prior to his coming to London, although he could remember having been in Boulogne for perhaps two days. He had become clear as to his immediate environment, but found difficulty in concentrating his mind on any topic. He said he had had visions of the Messines Ridge on going to sleep, and he was not quite sure whether he dreamed that he was there, or that he felt that he was there before actually going to sleep. There was absolutely no anxiety in these dreams, nor in the daytime, and no "nervousness" at any time. There were no neurological signs, but his eyes could not be examined on account of the intense photophobia from which he suffered.

He told of a recurrent dream which he had had for a good many nights, although it had not been present for the last two nights. The dream was as follows: His guns were being fired by creatures having the bodies of frogs and the heads of Bairnsfather's caricatures. These creatures did everything wrong and paid no attention to his orders, and he felt much annoyed by his inability to set things right. In the first dream they had the guns pointed backwards toward the British lines. In later dreams they were turning the treads from left to right instead of forward. Finally the creatures had the guns pointed toward the enemy, but did not fire them, simply stood there. The affect in all these dreams was the same, namely, annoyance at the inability to get his orders obeyed. It seemed that the men either did not hear, or paid no attention.

A superficial analysis of this dream was easily made, showing that the details were a jumble of ideas in his mind while on duty at Messines. Near his battery there was a pool full of frogs. German shells used to drop in this pond, after which frogs and slime would rain all around them, which was very annoying.

The Bairnsfather pictures he was very fond of, and had the walls of his dugout covered with them. The men not hearing them made him think of the frogs again. They used to croak very frequently. One of the sergeants had the name of "Brick," and there was a joke in the battery that one of the frogs had called out "Brick, Brick," and the sergeant had answered. An hour before the concussion, this sergeant, of whom the patient was fond, was wounded in the ear.

This is a typical fatigue dream, in which the task of the day is presented as something that is annoyingly impossible to complete, wherein the distortions from the actual situation are the result of other annoyances being included, tending to make the confusion and the impossibility of putting through the work all the greater. After these recurrent dreams he had an isolated one that was again a distortion of another difficulty at the front. For the last three weeks while on duty he had had trouble in getting up his ammunition and rations. In the dream he discovered one of the nurses at the hospital in which he was in London, trying to bring a box of tea into his room. She was having a hard time of it and could not succeed. He wanted to help her, but could not get to the door. He felt that the nurse was trying to bring him rations.

Nine days later I saw him again, at which time he felt very much better. His sight was still poor, particularly on the left, so he said. It was hard to believe that this was a neurotic difficulty for he burned his fingers slightly in lighting a cigarette. There was little ataxia in his movements. Speech had become quicker, but was still high pitched. It was also possible to detect an occasional defect, as when he said "t" for "th," and sometimes "d" for "l." His eye-grounds had been examined and found normal, but his visual fields had not been tested on account of the photophobia. He had received a letter from his captain giving the details of his accident and was astounded to learn that at least three days were gone from his memory.

The attitude of this patient toward the war and fighting was in marked contrast to that of the anxiety cases who are either consciously aware of their resistance to returning to the front, or exhibit this resistance in their dreams. The patient was anxious to return to duty because he had been promised the command of a battery that was to be sent to Italy. As he had never taken part in any mountain operations, this prospect was most attractive to him. His unconscious desire to take up this work is illustrated in the following dream, where difficulties are surmounted or made ridiculous. This dream occurred about a week after the last one quoted, and in the interval he had had none, or remembered none on waking. The dream is as follows: He was training men for Italy at Aldershot, and decided to take his men to a hilly country as that would be more like Italy. He therefore moved his battery to Devonshire and the men worked splendidly, so that he was proud of them. He made them bivouac out the first night, however, and they all caught cold in their left eyes (the patient's vision was poorer in the left eye). He despised the men for their softness, but realized that it was partly his fault and felt a little ashamed. Then the thought suddenly came to him that they would no longer need to close their left eyes when they sighted the guns, and he laughed aloud at the thought of it. He awoke laughing. That the patient in this dream disposed of the only symptom he was aware of which could prevent the assumption of his new duties, is too obvious to require further comment.

The following case illustrates another concussion in a normal individual in whom there had been a short period of fatigue prior to the accident, and possibly related to that, a brief development of anxiety symptoms after the accident.

CASE XIV. The patient is a ruggedly built officer about 30, who took out his commission at the beginning of 1916 and went to France at the beginning of 1917. Nothing indicating any abnormality could be discovered in his mental make-up during a brief examination. In his first exposure to shell fire he was frightened, but soon acquired the ability of gauging the direction of the shells, after which he had no fear whatever. The sight of bloodshed gave him no disabling symptoms, but he knew very well what they were, as he said he had seen many soldiers who had been incapacitated by horror. He fought for several months without any particular incident, and enjoyed the life. In May he was, with others, holding a salient for three days under terrible fire. The trenches had just been taken, both flanks were exposed and the enemy was making every effort to wipe out this advanced line. They had not had time to make any dugouts and so there was practically no protection from shells. On the third day only six out of twenty officers were left. About 11 in the morning the patient was buried and unconscious for a time.

On recovering consciousness he felt shaky and was "jumpy," but carried on because there were so few officers left. His mind was hazy and he wondered in a dazed sort of way how long he would be able to keep going, but was determined not to give up. He lost his ability to gauge the direction of the shells, and all the afternoon felt that the Germans were aiming directly at him. This is of course a definite symptom of the anxiety state, but not one from which recovery could not have been made if he had been relieved from duty before being exposed to further strain or accident.

About 6 o'clock that evening he was buried again and awoke six or seven hours later in a casualty clearing station, with a terrible headache, and incoherent. For the next two or three weeks he was conscious and unconscious off and on, and could talk very little as the words seemed to stick in his throat. His head ached, and he felt confused and was dizzy whenever he sat up in bed. From the fourth to the twelfth day he had a fever that went as high as 103° and 104°. When this left him, his recovery began and went steadily forward. When I saw him some six weeks after the concussion, he was able to sit up and talk a little. His speech was slow, in isolated phrases, and suggested a word-finding difficulty, with occasional wrong use of words, such as when he said to me as I took my leave: "Much obliged to meet you," a mistake of which he did not seem to be aware. Headaches were still present, coming on as a rule about 8 at night and keeping him awake half the night so that in the morning he would feel very dull. Some nights, however, he had no headache at all. Noises were very unpleasant to him and he started at every sudden sound, but without any trace of fear.

He confessed that his memory was still treacherous, and was hazy, particularly for the period of time he had spent in the hospital in France, and he still had some difficulty in concentration. He said that at first he had slept very little, and that when he did sleep his rest was disturbed by nightmares of being under bombardment in which every shell was coming at him. After a month the dreams became infrequent, and when he would awake a realization of his surroundings always made him perfectly comfortable, and he said that he had never had any fear whatever during the day.

In this case we have a clinical picture which is almost purely that of concussion, the only features of an anxiety neurosis being the trouble a few hours prior to the second concussion when he felt that the shells were coming directly at him, and nightmares lasting for a month or six weeks, with similar content.

Following the concussion, however, there were no diurnal symptoms whatever that could not be traced directly to the concussion. It was interesting that, unlike the neurotic patient, he talked spontaneously not at all of himself, and when personal questions were asked, replied to them briefly and then passed to some external subject.

The following cases illustrate the aggravation of anxiety symptoms by concussion in patients in whom the neurotic manifestations were already marked:

CASE XV. The patient is a sergeant of the regular army, aged 30, who denied having any definite nervous trouble prior to the war. He was afraid of the dark as a child, however, and had night terrors at this time. He has always had a fear of falling, and a slight feeling of faintness on going down in an elevator into the underground railway, or would begin to feel faint when in an underground train for any length of time, a symptom which he attributed to bad air. As a small boy he was not particularly mischievous, but became more one of the crowd after he had been a few years at school. He was also as a boy very shy with girls, and recovered less from that difficulty as he grew older than he did in respect to his sociability with men. He was engaged for three years, and married at 21, and there was apparently no reason for this long engagement. He claimed, however, that his married life had been very happy. He was eight years in the army before the war began, and acted as sergeant practically all the time, a work which he enjoyed greatly and in which he was quite efficient. He went to France with the first expeditionary force and remained there for eleven months. For a couple of days he was nervous about the shells, then got used to them and enjoyed the fighting hugely. He was extremely expert with the bayonet, having previously been an instructor in the use of that weapon, and derived considerable satisfaction from his success with it. After fighting nearly a year, he became tired and depressed and didn't care what happened particularly, but slept well and had absolutely no fear. Then suddenly he was wounded at the base of the spine and through the right lung with machine-gun bullets. The former was not particularly serious, but the latter was, for he lost a good deal of blood and had a haemothorax for many months. He was invalided home to England and was a long time in bed. During this period he felt fatigued and had many dreams at night of fighting. These were not dreams associated with fear, but more of the fatigue type, in which he was ceaselessly fighting without relief, and would awake in the morning tired from his efforts.

His convalescence was rather slow. For a long time he had difficulty in talking on account of his weakness and shortness of breath. After being in the hospital and on leave for five months he rejoined the army, although he still felt far from well. He was put on light duty, but this included drilling where he had to shout at his men, and he discovered that these efforts resulted in his spitting up blood. This not only alarmed him, but made him feel that he was being unwisely and unfairly treated in being placed on duty before he had completely recovered. This attitude was considerably accentuated by his being ordered a month later to return to France. He was sent to the Ypres section where his trenches were five hundred yards from the Germans, so that there was no possibility of any hand to hand fighting. He felt there was little justice in the system that could send an invalid into this terrible situation, and resentment was strong within him. He settled down into the routine, however, and ceased to think so much about this, although he became speedily very fatigued and fearful of the shells. These symptoms increased steadily and by the end of three months he had got to the point where he had very little sleep and wished fervently that some shell would take him out of his misery. Then one night he was buried and was under the earth for three-quarters of an hour. He came to some days later with practically no memory at all; in fact, all he knew was his own name. Consciousness apparently was coming and going for some time, and he was very hazy as to his movements for nearly two months. Although his memory steadily improved he had difficulty in concentration for at least six months. At first he could not speak at all; then for a month he would whisper, and when he recovered his voice he stammered for several months. Among his first memories were hallucinations of fighting, with great fear, which occurred during the day, and constant nightmares, many of them being of bayoneted or bombarded. The fear in these dreams was never of being wounded but always of being killed.

For many months he got not much more than an hour's sleep on any night, but after seven months of hospital treatment the dreams became somewhat less frequent and his quota of sleep rose to four hours a night. Headaches were most troublesome, being constant for the first month or so, and after that a frequent result of nightmare, as he would awake from one of his dreams in terror, and with a frightful pain in his head which might last for hours. He talked much in his sleep, and on awaking his head often felt very full, with a swimming, giddy sensation. During many months he lay awake at night for hours together, thinking of the war and imagining that he was in action.

He also had other, not so usual, symptoms, such as a feeling of nausea, difficulty in beginning to pass urine, and extreme constipation. He was subject to marked trembling. His head for many months shook almost constantly and he had also marked tremors of the legs. After he had been in the hospital for two months, an attempt was made to get him out of bed, but his legs trembled so violently and were so weak that he could not stand,

and any effort to make him walk resulted merely in very exaggerated movements of his legs.  When put back in bed his legs
would shake so violently that the bed trembled.  When put into
a wheel-chair his calf muscles were in such constant tremor that
the whole chair shook.

After some months the patient exhibited few signs of recovery
under the ordinary treatment of rest, and it became evident that
there was a definite reason for this.  He had an unusual depression.  He felt not only that he was not going to get well, but that
he did not wish to recover.  Visits from his wife made no impression on him.  He had no desire to see any friends and did
not care whether they were alive or dead.  In fact, this symptom
was so strong that when he heard of the death of his son, aged
4 years, he had difficulty in realizing it, and was not greatly impressed.  For several months he did not care about either the
success or failure of the war, although that was the first interest
to return.  It developed that the basis of this depression was his
feeling of resentment at the government and the country that
sent him back to fight after he had already done his duty; he had
suffered severely and was still an invalid.  He complained frequently of the way in which a "British subject is treated,"
mentioning his own experiences and his having frequently seen
men shot for suspected cowardice.  He thought that they, too,
were not treated as "British subjects" should be.  He confessed
to worrying about these incidents constantly, and that these
ideas were always in his mind when he returned to France the
second time.  The mechanism of this depression apparently was
that with this resentment contact with his fellows was broken.
He had no ambition to renew it, and consequently was an isolated
being for whom no one cared.  It is typical of the ready response
to treatment which the war neuroses show that a little personal
attention and explanation as to the objects of examination, in
which he was led to take some interest, completely removed this
depression, so that he became bright, cheerful and anxious to
get well.  In the next few days, during which I had an opportunity of seeing him, the recovery from many of these symptoms
was remarkable.  For one thing, he got so that he could walk

fairly well, and he was perfectly confident that he would soon be entirely recovered.

CASE XVI. The patient is a man of 45, very happily married for twenty years, who had been an efficient plumber with his own shop for many years. His make-up seems to have been unusually normal. At the beginning of the war he did not enlist because he was responsible for the maintenance of his family. When the first Zeppelin came over London, however, he felt that he could remain out of the war no longer and joined up, although it involved closing his business. He adapted himself well to the training, and then went to France, where he acted as senior sapper for 130 days. He enjoyed this work greatly, as he had a good gang of men under him and was able to do most effective work. He felt sorry for the wounded and the killed, but it did not upset him. Three weeks before the end of his stay in France his working party was spotted, and most of the men were killed by shells. Up to this time he said he had not felt overworked, but after it the war got on his nerves. The sight of the dead horrified him. He felt as if all the shells were coming at him, and was "jumpy" at every explosion. His sleep was poor and he began to have bad dreams. He became quite hopeless of being able to continue indefinitely, and wished that he might be killed. For three days he had such a headache that he was not able to hold his head up except when actively busy. Then a heavy high explosive shell buried him. It exploded so close that his hair and eyebrows were burned off. He remembered nothing of it, but was told that he must have fought his way up through the loose earth because his head and arms showed above ground. When the rescue party dug him out and brought him to the hospital, it was found that he had such a severe bruise on his buttocks that the doctor told him he would never walk again. This concussion took place on July 1, 1916. On July 7, he was taken to a hospital in London, and his memories begin again from his stay in that hospital. He knows he was conscious before reaching England but can recall nothing of the time. He could not talk without great effort in getting a word "off his chest," a difficulty which persisted for the better part of a year when he was at all excited. He was at first very deaf, and still is hard of hearing, although this has improved greatly. (Probably middle ear trouble.) He was so weak that he could not raise his eyes, and was short of breath, a symptom which was still present when I examined him in June, 1917. His legs were full of pain, and it was some months before he could walk. The pain, although greatly lessened in degree, persisted for a year. All these symptoms, except the weakness in the legs, he ascribed to the exposure to the noise and gases of the shells, which affected his eyes, his hearing and his lungs.

At first, in London, he could not recognize his wife, and could remember nothing about himself, but all his memory, except for the accident, came slowly back. Some forgetfulness as to the past was a persistent symptom. During the daytime he was constantly "jumpy," and trembling all over, although he felt no fear. In fact, the only diurnal fears he had were when a Zeppelin raid occurred and bombs fell in the immediate neighbourhood of the hospital, or when thunder-storms occurred. Also if he were left alone for a time, figures of Germans would begin to appear on the wall and he would become frightened. As he grew stronger and was able to move in a chair, he would get out of the room and join others when any of these visions occurred. He also suffered from hypnagogic hallucinations of Germans, sometimes with, sometimes without fear. Bad dreams, which were worse than any that he had at the front, began in the hospital. These, during the following year, gradually decreased, but were still occasionally present a year after the concussion. He could tell when they were going to come by a thumping in his head before going to sleep. The content of these was purely of fearful incidents in France. But later he began to dream of bombardment without fear.

He exhibited a splendid spirit. He blamed no one, and thought he simply had had bad luck. When it was suggested that he ought perhaps to have been given leave he scoffed at the idea, because the sappers were short-handed at the time. He was very anxious to get well and seemed to be improving rapidly in spite of having a high blood-pressure.

# CHAPTFR VII

## TREATMENT OF ANXIETY STATES

THE treatment of the anxiety states, although effective in an astonishingly large number of cases when intelligently pursued, is nevertheless not such a simple affair that the physician can be guided by any rule of thumb in his procedure. As has been stated, the symptoms of the neurosis (no matter what fundamental physical factors there may have been) seem invariably to be determined psychologically. Plainly then, the psychological effect of every therapeutic measure must be considered. In this report the etiological factors have been given prominence because it seems that the treatment of the anxiety cases must be individual, and must, in every instance, be aimed at the removal of the effect of each cause. It cannot be too strongly urged that consistent plans of treatment should be followed, as would readily be admitted by all who have been interested in the treatment of neurotics during times of peace. There is, therefore, nothing more inimical to the interests of the patient (or of the army, in the long run) than a frequent transfer of these patients from one hospital to another, where different theories are held as to the cause of the trouble, or where notes do not accompany the patients, giving an outline of what has already been accomplished or attempted.

At the outset, every patient, once a diagnosis is made (and it should be made speedily), ought to be removed as quickly as possible to a quiet environment. It must be borne in mind constantly that a highly important factor in every case is the conscious or unconscious desire to get away from the fighting. Not unnaturally then, symptoms tend to be aggravated by mere removal from the line and having the patient placed under the observation of a physician, because the worse impression the patient makes, the longer is his absence from the trenches apt to be. Consequently, we obtain the history from many patients of symptoms becoming very much greater as soon as they arrive in a hospital. (Merely coming under observation is not the only reason for this exaggeration of symptoms.) Since the soldier is incompetent to fight, he must be in a hospital, but once there, he should be protected during this period from every possible excitement that is liable to increase his symptoms. The stay in any hospital which is under shell fire, near parade grounds, or filled with wounded men, should therefore be cut down to the minimum. On the other hand, if the patient be taken too far from the firing line, if he be sent over seas, for instance, he is likely to develop an idea of permanent absence from his duties that may stand in the way of a complete recovery. Ideally, therefore, we should seek to place these men in a hospital quietly situated in the same country where the fighting is in progress.

The treatment at first should be purely symptomatic. Every patient suffers more or less from fatigue, and little is gained by psychological treatment in one who is suffering from such a definitely physical disability as severe fatigue. The first effort should be to give the patient absolute rest in bed and produce sleep in as normal a way as possible. The Weir Mitchell type of treatment is of value with some cases, but if the patient is subject to fear when left alone, isolation can by no possibility lead to any improvement in his condition. Some idea of the individual difficulties must therefore be gained at once. The question of producing sleep is also one concerning which no general rule can be laid down. Although there is nothing worse for these patients than the indiscriminate and constant use of sedatives, they may nevertheless be of great value if properly administered. A good method is to give sufficient dosage of whatever drug seems to be indicated to produce sleep the first night when treatment is begun. The patient should be kept as quiet as possible during the following day, and an effort be made to produce sleep the next night in a more normal manner, that is, by the use of baths, packs, etc. Mild suggestion may be of considerable value at this stage. In practical experience the most potent influence in suggestion seems to be the general morale and attitude of a hospital as a whole. It is a striking fact that in those hospitals where reliance is placed chiefly on drugs there is a constant difficulty met with in combating insomnia, whereas the difficulties are much less in those institutions where drugs are largely taboo. If, on the second night, no sleep is obtained by hydrotherapeutic methods or suggestion, a milder dosage of a hypnotic may be effective, and for this a placebo may be later substituted.

The above statements refer to the acute stage where genuine fatigue is undoubtedly present. It must be borne in mind that fatigue, as such, is a condition which is readily and rather speedily recovered from simply through rest. Consequently the period during which the patient is kept isolated and no demands are made for him to exert himself in the slightest degree, should be kept as brief as possible. If this is not done, a condition of invalidism is fostered. Just how long this period should be is a matter which must be settled individually, but as a general rule one might say that the patient should not be left without any demands being made for cooperation on his part in the treatment for longer than one or two weeks. This is, however, rather a guess, inasmuch as I have not had an opportunity of seeing many of these cases immediately after they have been in the trenches. It is of course obvious that when concussion of any severity has occurred, a very much longer period of rest is indicated, as we know even from civilian experience that nothing is more inimical to the welfare of one suffering from physical injury to the brain than fatigue. Complete and prolonged rest for these cases is therefore obligatory. At present we have no drugs that combat fatigue of the central nervous system directly. If further study of these cases reveals the chemical nature of this disease, we might hope to find some antidote for it that would materially reduce the period of rest required. Further than that, we might even hope that the same remedy would prevent the steady increase of the cumulative effects of the fatigue that we see in the trenches, and thus prevent many neuroses from developing beyond the initial stages, where fatigue dominates the clinical picture.

Proceeding along the lines of symptomatic treatment, the next stage should be to combat the patient's most obvious subjective difficulties, namely, the fear of war and the obsessions with thought of its horrors. These can best be met acutely by distraction in one form or another. The patient should be given a common sense talk and assured of two things: The first is that he is going to get well, since he has been removed temporarily from the influences which caused his breakdown, and that this recovery will be greatly facilitated by his active cooperation. The second is that he is now under medical control and that he need have no fear of being ordered to do anything that will not be to the advantage of his health, that there is no possibility of his being sent back to the line until he is completely well, but that, on the other hand, because his disease is curable, he will, of course, have to return eventually. In other words, an effort must be made to produce a state of mind wherein he is willing to forget the war, for the time being, without fostering the idea that he is out of it for good. It is not enough for the patient merely to be willing to forget. Active efforts must be made to distract his mind. His environment should therefore be made as nearly that of civilian life as is possible and practicable. This does not mean that uniforms should be abandoned. The men are still in the army, and should not be given such a suggestion as to leaving the service. Rigorous military discipline, however, should be relaxed, and the artificial social distinctions between different ranks reduced to a minimum. A medical man, for instance, who cannot forget that he has the rank of major, is bound to make a pitiful failure in his efforts to treat a subaltern.

Occupation of some kind should invariably be given, but never according to any hard and fast rules. A game of cards may be all the man can stand at first, perhaps it will be only a very small amount of light reading. He can progress from this to the less violent out-of-door games, and as his strength increases, be given something more productive. For this reason, well equipped workshops are invaluable, particularly for pri-

vates and non-commissioned officers. A course of study is sometimes of considerable value for an officer whose interests are
naturally in an intellectual field. The objects of these occupations are two-fold, being first, to distract the man's mind from
the worries that had so much to do in the establishment of his
neurosis, and secondly, to give him that confidence in himself
which is often painfully lacking, and which can be re-established
only by the patient's actually achieving something. The pre-
scribing of occupations should always be directly under the
control of the physician in charge of the case, whose duty it is to
note the exact effect which the occupation has on the patient,
and to vary its nature or aim accordingly. Much harm is frequently done by advising some exertion which fatigues him un-
duly, and convinces him that he has some terrible weakness.
The consequent discouragement may be extreme, and for a long
time stand in the way of any improvement. Every patient
should therefore be examined with great frequency, particularly
at the beginning of any occupation treatment. The granting of
leave from the hospital for a few hours, or for a week-end, if
judiciously used, may help a patient considerably. He is thrown
on his own resources to a greater extent than when in the hospital
environment, and consequently he has a much greater feeling of
achievement and greater pleasure from this than from any intra-
mural entertainment. As practically all those who suffer from
anxiety neuroses are impotent, at least in the acuter stages,
sexual indiscretions do not need to be borne in mind, when leave
is granted, so constantly as they do when the patients are suffering from other forms of disability. In fact, feminine companion-
ship is an excellent form of distraction to the soldier who has
been for many months in a purely military environment.

The treatment so far outlined is essentially environmental, and
aims at combating the symptoms in a superficial way. In most
cases it will be successful in removing all or most of the obvious
symptoms. There remains, however, the fundamental difficulty
which has so much to do with the development of the neurosis,
namely, the antagonism to the duties forced on the soldier, and
often to war in general. These can be eradicated *only* by the

patient gaining some psychological understanding of the origin and nature of his symptoms. Occasionally one meets with an officer who is sufficiently intelligent to understand the situation without any outside help, and who is capable of taking himself in hand and combating these tendencies alone. This, however, is rare.

On the other hand, those who have experienced the great difficulties to be met with in civilian practice, in getting patients to understand themselves, will be delighted with the ease with which the sufferers from war neuroses are capable of grasping the psychology of their disease and making use of their knowledge. This is, of course, not unnatural, considering that we deal here with men who are, relatively speaking, quite normal, and with situations that are essentially simple. In a few talks a patient can be led to see how the war sublimation, which has been outlined, has broken down, and how it was that he therefore developed the tendency to think of himself rather than of the needs of the army and of the country, and so became a prey to fear and horror.

When once the patient sees that his disinclination to return to the front is essentially a selfish desire to avoid his responsibility as a citizen, he is in a position to decide quite consciously whether he wishes to be a slacker or to assume his share of the country's burden. If he has the right stuff in him, he becomes ashamed of his symptoms and begins to control them quite speedily. He is soon eager to take some part in the struggle, and if he is given light duty which does not make too great a demand on his capacity, this capacity grows, and with it a desire to return to the field of active operations appears. Probably nothing is gained by an attempt to send a man back to the firing line who does not spontaneously wish to be there. Each patient has learned that the development of certain symptoms will cause his removal from the trenches, and if he consciously desires to be out of them he will make little effort to combat their redevelopment.

Even when this type of analysis is attempted, reliance should not be placed on it alone. It cannot be too constantly borne in mind that one of the greatest difficulties from which these neurotics suffer is a lack of complete rapport with their fellows. Many of them feel (with some justice) that they have been ill-treated, and a feeling of responsibility toward the State is difficult to foster in an individual who feels that the State has no regard for him. For this reason a demonstration of personal interest in the patient may be of great value (Case XV is an example of this). The physician must therefore learn to have a keen sympathy for the patient as an individual, but never to have any sympathy whatever for the patient's symptoms as such. This is not an easy attitude to acquire, and is probably the reason why few physicians who are not trained psychiatrists are successful in treating the war neuroses.

As has been said before, there is a tendency present, particularly among those having had a definite neurotic history before the war, to develop neurotic troubles of the civilian type when convalescence from an anxiety state is achieved. It is not within the provinces of this report to enter into the treatment of these complicating neuroses, inasmuch as they are essentially peace disturbances. In so far, however, as they are determined by unconscious resistance to active service, they are amenable to treatment in a greater degree than are similar neuroses of civilian life, for this is, psychologically speaking, a simpler situation than that which, as a rule, precipitates a neurosis in a civilian.

# CHAPTER VIII

## CONVERSION HYSTERIAS

THE conversion hysterias do not require so protracted a discussion as it has seemed wise to devote to the anxiety cases. Although in absolute numbers they are more frequent in occurrence than pure anxiety states, yet they are so much simpler in mechanism that it is less difficult to understand them and to treat them. Moreover, much of what has already been said as to fatigue and dissatisfaction with active service may be applied directly in discussing the conversion hysterias, provided one remembers that, although these factors operate in the two conditions alike, their development is much less extensive in the cases of conversion hysteria.

These may be defined as neuroses in which there is an alteration or dissociation of consciousness regarding some physical function. The term *"Conversion Hysteria"* is used, because an idea is carried over into a physical symptom. These cases are confined almost entirely to privates and non-commissioned officers, the reason for which will be discussed later. The purely hysterical manifestations are apt to be accompanied by mild anxiety symptoms; occasionally the latter are severe.

The symptomatology is extremely varied, although there have been no symptoms described in the war cases, so far as I know, which have not been well known in times of peace. Even a brief study convinces one that the more important and frequent symptoms are those which obviously provide the patient with a relief from active service. Mutism is the commonest, apparently. Aphonia as a preliminary symptom is rarer, but it often develops as a stage of recovery from mutism, as does stammering. Deafness is fairly frequent. After the speech group, motor disturbances are the most important.   These include monoplegias and paraplegias or pareses; tics, spasms and contractures are not unusual.   Tremors are usually a complication of an anxiety state, and it is quite frequent to find gait disturbances such as have been described in connexion with the anxieties.   For instance one sees an initial and not very severe anxiety state in a private develop into a gait disturbance that is unaccompanied by any emotional trouble.   Spasticity of the legs is also a rare symptom, except as a complication or result of an anxiety state. Hyperaesthesias may occur alone.   Paraesthesia and anaesthesia usually accompany hysterical symptoms.   Blindness and amblyopia are not very common.   Disorders of smell and taste are still rarer.

*Clinical Course.*   What has been said as to the make-up in connexion with the anxiety states applies also to the hysterical group, but with the latter complete normality seems to be more frequent.   The adaptation to training may or may not be good; naturally those who adapt themselves well are less likely to develop symptoms.   Fatigue is, as a rule, the first symptom that can be discovered, but it is almost never so severe as in the anxiety cases.   Its symptoms are therefore not so well marked. There is little sleeplessness, and rarely nightmares, in the purely hysterical case.   More frequently one gets a history of diurnal dissatisfaction.   As a rule, there is fear, with much less "jumpiness" than is met with among officers.   There is almost always some weariness and a distinct antagonism to the fighting.   The patient is rarely subjected to the mental conflicts that are so distinctive of the prodromal anxiety state in officers, because the men who develop hysterical symptoms are privates whose ideals are not so high, and who do not have to make decisions for themselves.   Their responsibilities begin and end with obedience to orders.   And it is the duty of the officers to put courage into them, not for them to develop and maintain it themselves.   Not unnaturally then, we find these men seeking to gain release from the situation they dislike in a way which is incompatible with the higher standards of the officers.   They look for some valid excuse for absence from the firing line, and so, almost universally, hope to be wounded in some way that will incapacitate them from active service.  I have found either this wish for a "Blighty one," or else thoughts of some physical disease, in the history of every hysterical case, except one, that I had an opportunity of examining.  The exceptional patient did not seem sufficiently intelligent to give an accurate history.  Occasionally the antagonism to fighting is the direct outcome of physical accident or disease which removes the soldier from the trenches. The wish that develops is then that he may not have to return.

The attitude of antagonism with some idea of release constitutes the background of the hysteria.  Then something happens which is the occasion for the development of definite symptoms.  A frequent cause is concussion which may or may not be severe.  Case XV, the sergeant who was exhausted and had been worried about his inability to shout without spitting up blood, and therefore had his attention directed to his voice, is an example in point.  After his concussion and return to consciousness he was mute, following that, aphonic, and then stammered. A not infrequent symptom is anaesthesia at the area of some slight injury which is received at the time of concussion.  Not unnaturally burial without concussion is a highly frequent precipitating factor.  It is not improbable that the overstrung soldier imagines that he is about to be killed when the shell explodes close to him, and this emotional shock upsets his mind sufficiently to cause that disturbance of consciousness which we term hysteria.  As with the anxiety cases, the infliction of an actual wound does not at the time precipitate hysterical symptoms, but these very often develop later when the private who does not wish to fight is convalescing physically from his wound. The subjective symptoms are apt to be continued indefinitely in a hysterical way, that is, the pain or disability may not be recovered from, although there may be complete healing at the site of injury.  Monoplegias or spasticities are common symptoms with this etiology.  Torticollis may also occur in this way. It is not difficult to reconstruct the original history of these cases. There is, while a soldier is still in the trenches, the usual wish to be away from the distasteful employment.  This wish reaches its fulfilment when a disabling wound is received, a situation which is quite satisfactory so long as the injury continues to be disabling. Once recovery sets in, however, the prospect of returning to the trenches is plainly before the eyes of the soldier. Under these circumstances, while he is both consciously and unconsciously loth to leave the comfortable position in which he finds himself, he naturally pays considerable attention to the pain or disability that is a direct outcome of his wound. This attention, backed by his wish for the symptoms to be permanent, convinces him that there is no improvement in any respect that is to him subjectively obvious. Consequently his consciousness gradually adapts itself to the disability until it is incapable of conceiving the idea of true recovery. The patient, therefore, whose head has been bandaged over to one side with a wound in the neck, continues to hold his head in that position in spite of the fact that there is no real contracture of scar tissue. Similarly the man whose arm may have been put up in a sling finds when the sling is removed that all power is gone from the arm, or the limb which has been held in a certain position to avoid pain on movement is retained spastically in that position. As may be readily understood, medical officers in many cases unthinkingly suggest disabilities to these patients by the method of their examination or the nature of their questions. Apart from the presence of objective symptoms, the patient may be in a normal mental state. He is usually untroubled by any anxiety, is not easily fatigued, and his behaviour is that of any wounded man, that is to say it is quite normal.

As long as war is in progress and return to the front is imminent the patient prefers (unconsciously at least) to retain his disability rather than to face the perils and discomforts of trench life. Consequently these symptoms, when not treated, persist as a rule indefinitely. Occasionally through some accident the patient discovers that the function, which he thought he had lost, is still present. This usually occurs under the stimulus of some sudden emotion. It is, of course, one thing for an outsider to observe a man using a paralyzed arm and another thing for the patient himself to be aware of it. This is only to be expected when we consider that one of the most fundamental characteristics of a hysterical symptom is that consciousness, and therefore awareness, as to the function in question is lost. The patients who recover spontaneously, therefore, by making such observations themselves are rare. On the other hand, owing probably to the simplicity of the mental mechanisms involved, treatment is as a rule a very simple matter and frequently successful in a dramatic and permanent way. Once the disability has been recovered from, the patient is in a much more normal state than is a man suffering from anxiety whose obvious symptoms have disappeared.

The diagnosis of these conversion hysterias is not so simple a matter as that of the anxiety states. Any competent neurologist should of course be able by the usual methods to make speedy and accurate discrimination between organic and functional loss. When the two are combined, however, the problem becomes somewhat more difficult. Hysterical anaesthesia, for instance, may occur with, but have a wider distribution than, that of a pure nerve injury. The latter may be overlapped by the former and lead the physician to believe that he is dealing with a purely hysterical condition. A final diagnosis may therefore be made, only after treatment instituted on purely functional lines has been successful, and has reduced the disability to its legitimately organic distribution. Quite the most difficult problem, however, is to differentiate a conversion hysteria from malingering. As I have had little opportunity to see cases of malingering as they are presented at the front, I am unable to say much on this topic that is not second-hand. Some workers rely largely on the suggestibility of the hysterical patient as a diagnostic criterion. Occasionally one meets with a physician who goes so far as to state that no patient who is not hypnotizable has a true hysteria, and therefore must be malingering. As the individual capacity to hypnotize varies greatly from man to man this is probably a rather unsafe rule. Again, if one relies on the impression which the personality of the patient makes on the physician error is apt to be frequent. The true malingerer is frequently, if not always, a psychopath. Again it may require a rather exhaustive study

to determine whether the symptoms are produced on the basis
of a conscious or an unconscious wish, which is essentially the
difference in etiology between malingering and hysteria.  Probably the safer guide is the history of onset.  One should inquire, therefore, as to the mental attitude of the patient before
the onset of the symptoms.  In a true hysterical case an admission is apt to be made as to the breaking down of adaptation to
warfare and the consequent wish to be rid of it all, particularly
the wish for an incapacitating wound.  The malingerer is not apt
to reveal the history because the symptom represents this wish
to him quite consciously.  The hysteric, on the other hand, because there has been an unconscious motivation, does not see the
connexion between his previous desire to be incapacitated and
the symptom his malady presents.  He is, therefore, more apt
to be frank in the matter.  In another respect the history may be
of importance, I imagine.  In all the cases, which I have had an
opportunity of examining, whose symptoms arose while in the
trenches, there was a history either of concussion or of definite
precipitating cause, the immediate result of which was some disturbance of consciousness, no matter how slight.  Frequently it
amounted to no more than the patient being dazed for a few
minutes and finding himself with the hysterical symptom, when
he became quite clear again.  As the opinion of the physician on
this matter when delivered to a court martial may mean life or
death for the soldier I would prefer to leave this last diagnostic
criterion as a suggestion until such time as further experience
may show whether the phenomenon in question is universal
or not.

The prognosis in these cases depends on a number of factors.
An important one is naturally the mental make-up of the patient.
An individual who has a definite psycho-neurotic make-up is
prone to develop symptoms, to cling to them more tenaciously,
and to develop new ones if his original cause for removal from
the firing line is done away with.  The more normal soldiers, as
has been stated, are apt to keep their symptoms indefinitely until
appropriate treatment is instituted.  Once cured, they are delighted with the result and rarely suffer a relapse.  Inappropriate

treatment, however, is so ineffective that the opinion has grown up that it is useless to try to get these men back to the trenches. The experience gained in the better hospitals which are devoted to the care of the neuroses speaks distinctly against this, as they have sent a large proportion of their patients back to France, only a few of whom have relapsed.

Various types of treatment are in common use. The one which appeals most to the physician who has a military mind is discipline; and this is logical enough if the assumption be made that the symptoms are really under conscious control. If fear of punishment is greater than fear of the life in active service, the symptoms will naturally tend to disappear. On the other hand, the well-disciplined soldier has the habit of obeying developed to such an extent that he is highly suggestible to commands from those of superior rank. These two factors apparently account for the cures which result from this method of treatment. They are, however, few in number and not apt to be permanent. This can be easily explained psychologically if one bears in mind what has previously been reiterated as to the adaptation of the soldier. An all-essential factor in this adaptation is the feeling of unity with his group which the individual develops. Undue coercion—in fact any treatment which the patient may regard as unfair—is apt to weaken the bonds between the soldier and the army rather than to strengthen them; consequently although the symptoms may temporarily disappear, the wish for escape from military life is apt to be even stronger than it was before, so that a still firmer foundation for neurotic symptoms is built up. The application of electricity in various forms and of massage is highly popular and more often successful than disciplinary treatment. Its results, however, are dependent purely upon suggestion, and therefore open to the criticisms which will immediately be made of this method.

Naturally enough conversion hysterias arise on a background of extreme suggestibility. It is not surprising, therefore, that any form of suggestion—particularly hypnotism—is extraordinarily effective in the removal of the immediate symptoms. Moreover it does not serve to alienate the soldier from the army for which he has been fighting. On the other hand it has a grave defect psychologically in that it is aimed at the removal of symptoms rather than causes. To the uneducated soldier the symptom has come from nowhere and, if it is removed by the suggestion of electricity or the more direct suggestion of hypnosis, it leaves him through the agency of a miracle—consequently his mind is strongly imbued with the idea that such things can happen, with the not unnatural result that they do happen again. What should be aimed at is much more the training of the patient to control the workings of his mind, steadily combating the idea that there is anything miraculous or lawless about the functions of his body which have gone wrong. What is essentially re-education is, therefore, without any question the best method of treatment for the conversion hysterias. Those who are most successful in gaining permanent results begin as a rule with an introductory talk, when they explain to the patient the nature of the disease from which he suffers. They impress upon his mind the fact that his legs, for instance, are not really paralyzed but that he has simply forgotten how to use them and that he must learn to do so over again. An effort is made to make the soldier understand that this process is perfectly natural and that it will be quickly successful provided he makes the necessary effort. The next stage is to demonstrate that the function which is lost or disturbed is really not vitally affected. At this point suggestion or hypnotism may be of great value, provided that the patient be given immediately and convincingly the explanation that he has done these things rather than that the physician has accomplished them. Many of those whose treatment is most successful prefer to rely on some sort of trick in demonstrating the presence of the capacity which seems to be gone. It would be impossible to enumerate all these—in fact it is probably best to leave the choice of method to the natural ingenuity of the one who is responsible for the treatment. A few examples, however, may be given. One has already been cited in Case II, in which the patient who was deaf and dumb, was made to see in a mirror that he jumped when a sudden sound occurred behind his back. Patients who are mute or aphonic may be shown that all the movements of the lips, tongue and glottis which are necessary to produce speech have not been lost. The patient, for instance, may be able to whistle, to put his tongue in required positions, or to cough. In order to make the patient breathe evenly Captain McDowall has introduced the method of inducing the patient to inhale a cigarette, the smoke from which, if forcibly or irregularly expelled, is apt to be irritating and may produce a cough. Coughing of course involves the use of the vocal chords and produces a voiced sound. Any patient who can cough can also say "ah" and the training may begin from this point. That power is not lost from limbs may be demonstrated by the presence of reflexes, or of contractions elicited by electrical stimulation or by sudden movements that are made to prevent falling, etc. A means which is frequently effective is to induce passive movements while the operator actually does less and less in the way of movement until after a few trials the patient makes the motions without any aid from the operator at all. Where a swimming tank is available a demonstration of the ability to use the legs perfectly can be readily made in those patients who suffer from difficulties in walking. Apparently no matter how severe any gait disturbance may be there seems to be no interference with the function of the legs in swimming. Once it has been demonstrated that any function is not totally absent, it is the responsibility of the physician to see that constant practice is made and to insist on a steady increase in the extent and number of movements that are executed. When this treatment is patiently carried out improvement is apt to be rapid and the results permanent. The reason for the latter is that the patient has learned two things: first, that his symptom originated mainly in a lack of control, and secondly, that he has found a method of controlling symptoms when they do arise or tend to develop.

Many of these patients, of course, have personal difficulties which operate in connexion with the simple motivation, that has been discussed, in the production of, or maintenance of, symptoms. Many soldiers realize vaguely that their symptoms, although obvious in a physical way, are really mental in origin. The result of this is to produce in the uneducated man a belief that he is going insane. This is naturally a fear which he is apt to keep to himself, and one which is bound to increase his worry and therefore make his symptoms worse or more permanent unless he can have the situation carefully explained to him and this ridiculous fancy dispelled. It is therefore of first importance for the physician to establish friendly relationship with the patient and encourage him to bring his troubles to the consulting room for discussion and advice. Improvement when some quite simple personal problem has been cleared up is sometimes so rapid as to be startling. In connexion with this individual treatment one factor must not be lost sight of: the majority of the men who are now fighting in all the armies in Europe are essentially civilians. For the greater part of their lives therefore they have been accustomed to natural and friendly social contacts. In the army the demands of discipline necessitate much more artificiality, particularly in the relationship between officers and men. As a result the private soldier is very apt to feel a need for friendly advice such as he was able to receive in times of peace from his physician, employer or clergyman. Not unnaturally a feeling of isolation may grow up during his military life which operates to increase his dissatisfaction with the employment that is forced upon him. The private soldier is therefore extraordinarily affected for the better when any sympathy is shown him by a superior officer such as his physician is. Any hospital in which a minimum of stress is laid on military artificialities is incomparably more successful in the treatment of these cases than is one where military discipline is rigidly enforced, and, it may be added, a wise laxity in this regard tends to increase the respect which the private soldier feels for his superiors rather than to diminish it.

Any physician who has a reasonable fund of common sense and a natural interest in his patients is bound to be successful in the treatment of many of these cases. On the other hand, as has been said before, great care must be taken not to confuse sympathy for the patient with that sympathy for the patient's suffering which fosters a hypochondriacal tendency. For this reason the man who can best treat the war neuroses is he who has had years of experience in handling neurotic patients and has learned to be sympathetic with the sufferer as an individual and yet to be impatient with the symptoms as such.

After these general statements as to the causation, symptomatology and treatment of the conversion hysterias it may be well to quote a few illustrative cases.

CASE XVII. The patient is a lieutenant in the Royal Flying Corps, aged 23. His clinical history gives an excellent example of final symptoms representing a regression to a previous disability, which had occasioned him some worry. In make-up he was apparently an unusually normal individual who had at no time shown any neurotic tendencies and had a frank and open personality. He had supported himself from the age of 14, at which time his father died, had been successful in business, and had in addition found time to develop into quite an athlete, as well as to become socially popular with both sexes. He entered the army in the first year of the war, took well to his training and enjoyed the fighting keenly. For over a year he was in the infantry. About a year before the onset of his symptoms he was caught suddenly in a gas attack from which he suffered severely. He was in bed for some days and then, although he recovered rather quickly in other respects, had a severe tracheitis and laryngitis that persisted for weeks. Not unnaturally he was able to do no more than whisper for some time. As it happened, this disability was a considerable blow to the patient because he had always taken a considerable interest in his voice. He had been a good singer and was very proud of his ability to make his voice carry on the parade ground for a much greater distance than could his brother officers. When his voice returned he was much worried to find that any effort to shout caused it to become worse, after which his voice would be quite weak for some hours or days. On the first occasion when he was granted leave he went to London and consulted a laryngologist, who unfortunately told him that he would never be able to sing again. This was a distinct blow and he worried about it considerably, although this worry never was severe enough to incapacitate him as a soldier in the slightest degree. He continued to enjoy the life extremely.

As he was obviously fitted for that type of work he was transferred from the infantry to the Royal Flying Corps and soon became an expert airman. In the Spring of 1917 he one day went over the enemies' lines and made the necessary observations so quickly as to avoid attack. While returning he was shot at by the anti-aircraft guns. The shrapnel, so far as he was aware, although bursting thickly around him, did not hit him or his machine, but he considered it advisable to return to his own lines. As a matter of fact one of the wings of his machine had been hit and consequently weakened. The sudden strain thrown on this wing when he was landing caused it to break, so that he crashed to the ground. Careful inquiry failed to reveal any history of his feeling at all upset or nervous prior to the instant of this accident. As a matter of fact he was elated over his success. After striking the ground he was unconscious for three hours. When he came to he saw his servant in the distance and tried to attract his attention. Whether he attempted to shout and found his voice too weak or not he was unable to remember, as his memory was never entirely clear for the first few minutes after recovering consciousness. At any rate, it was some time before the servant came to him and when he did he found the patient unable to speak. It seems reasonable to suppose that with the concussion he received and the consequent mental confusion his mind harked back to the only physical trouble which he had ever known, namely, the disturbance of his voice that had worried him so much. He may have lived over in this brief period of confusion the previous accident when he was gassed. At any rate, he seems to have automatically begun to protect his voice as he had trained himself to do for the last year. This time, however, the effort of protection was so extreme as to be pathological and resulted in total disuse of his voice.

The concussion from which he suffered seems to have been mild in degree, for after a couple of days' rest he felt quite well physically. For two weeks he was in a hospital in France and then, as there was no improvement in his mutism, he was sent to England, where I saw him three weeks after the accident. In this hospital efforts were at once made to make him talk, and these speedily were successful in so far as he learned to whisper a few words.  He was soon able to whisper anything that he wished to say, although it seemed always to require a greater mental than physical effort.  By making him cough and then say "ah" he gained the use of the voiced sounds.  Another symptom then developed, namely, that of stammering.  It seemed as if he could bring himself to say not more than one or two words with one breath.  By training him to say two, three, four and then five letters of the alphabet in one expiration he was able to make considerable improvement in this.  Finally, under mild hypnosis that was practically nothing more than distraction, normal speech was attained that produced an even, uninterrupted repetition of the alphabet.  He was forced to apply this smoothness in utterance to his ordinary conversation at once, and did not relapse.  The next stage in his treatment was to get him to sing, and after a few weeks' practice he discovered that his singing voice was practically as good as ever it had been.  The total treatment lasted about six weeks, but would not have required so much time had the physician who was taking charge of it been able to see the patient every day.

The next case also illustrates a probable regression to a previous laryngitis with the production of mutism.

CASE XVIII.  The patient is a private, aged 26, who had a normal make-up apparently but was not sufficiently intelligent to answer all the questions concerning the minuter details of his mental life.  It was impossible to induce him to give any data as to his subjective experience—in fact he seemed to be one of those individuals who are totally incapable of any introspection.  Before his symptoms developed he had been fifteen months in France and had not received a scratch.  At first he had been in the Ypres section, and there had been sickened by the sight of wounds, did not like the idea of having to kill the Germans, and was frightened by the shells.  He got used to all these things, however, and then rather liked the warfare.  He was particularly proud of the work of the bombing squad of which he was a member.  He was able to give no history of exhaustion,

nervousness or bad dreams before his final accident. While at
Ypres he was gassed and laid up for a week. He had little re-
collection of what symptoms he showed at that time or of any
resemblance they might have to the ones he developed later. In
July, 1916, he was blown up by a shell which he could remember
seeing as it burst at his side. His companions told him that he
was blown into the air. He received a wound in the back and the
right arm and lost a great deal of blood. He was operated on
and came to only after several days. He then found himself
with a bad headache, dizzy, and with consciousness coming and
going for several days. The first time he was conscious it lasted
for only a few seconds. The next time a nurse was there who
spoke to him. He could not understand what she said and tried
to speak. He found he could not. This was possibly due either
to weakness or to aphasia which so many patients suffering from
concussion show for a short time. The patient was also deaf for
some days, and it is possible that not being able to hear any
sounds which he did make he developed the idea that he was
really dumb. For some time he was so numb all over that he
could not feel his wounds. This was possibly also a hysterical
symptom that was essentially a protective matter. At any rate,
he was mute from then on. He had difficulty in thinking for
several weeks. His memory for these first weeks was extremely
vague and he may have been subjected to some shocks during
this period which he later forgot. He was at this time in a
hospital that was subject to bombardment. And he remembers
that he was "jumpy" there, and fearful when anyone approached
him. Nightmares began which continued for a year with gradual
improvement. The setting of these dreams was always in France
with a constant content of being wounded and having a fear of
death, the latter fear predominating over any anxiety about
wounds. He said that in these first weeks he thought of the
fighting all the time and that when the acuity of his consciousness would lapse he would see the trenches and the enemy, but
did not have any hallucination of hearing.

The patient was treated in general hospitals for ten months
and showed no improvement whatever except in that his dreams

became somewhat less insistent. He was then transferred to a special hospital where improvement began at once and had continued steadily throughout the month that had elapsed before I examined him. He was then able to speak and make all the necessary voiced sounds, but suffered considerably from stammering and a distortion due to over-action of the lips and tongue. He could sing, however, with only an occasional stumbling.

As has been said, the patient was not able to give a fully intelligent account of his symptoms or mental state at different times. Any explanation as to psychological mechanisms of his mutism must therefore remain purely speculations. There can be no doubt that he suffered from a severe concussion and that the symptoms he showed on recovering consciousness—weakness, deafness and confusion—could be attributed directly to the physical effects of the concussion. Whether the dumbness was due to the weakness, the deafness, or was a direct product of a temporary aphasia it is impossible to say. Myers has suggested that mutism may be psychologically an outcome of stupor. Stupor is, he says, essentially a shutting out of the environment and, as speech is the chief means of communication which an individual has with his environment, it is not unnatural that mutism should survive and represent symbolically the lack of contact with his surroundings. As I have not had an opportunity of examining these cases at this stage I am not competent to criticize this view with any assurance. This would certainly be a natural type of mechanism and fits in well with what we know of stupors and hysterias in times of peace, but this applies to stupors that are functional and not organic in origin. In the case just quoted, for instance, the symptoms of an organic type are sufficiently evident to justify the belief that the unconsciousness from which he suffered was not at all functional but depended upon the concussion directly.

CASE XIX. The patient is a corporal who was apparently normal in mental make-up except for some shyness with the opposite sex. He went to France in May, 1915, after some months of training to which he adapted himself well. He was at once exposed to eighteen days of almost continuous bombardment. He was frightened at first, but got used to it, and settled down to his work quite satisfactorily. In September, 1915, the weather had been very bad and he got tired of the situation. He began to have bad dreams. Most of these were of the peace type of falling into a deep hole, but he also had nightmares of being shelled. His account of this period was rather indefinite. He admitted, however, that he was so tired of the situation he thought of committing suicide. .He also wished that a shell would give him an incapacitating wound or else kill him. He began to have pains in his head, arms and legs, and was feeling distinctly "groggy" when a gas attack came. He thinks he may have got a whiff of the gas; at any rate he felt giddy, but was able to pull off his mask for an instant and take a swallow of water. This made him feel a bit better and the gas having passed he came out of the dugout into the open air. He felt somewhat fatigued after this experience, however, and was much relieved when his company was ordered back that night. Once back to the lines, however, he got very shaky and finally collapsed, falling in a heap on a pile of straw. At the time·of this collapse he did not lose consciousness at all. From his own account and from notes made at the hospital to which he was immediately taken, it seems likely that he had an attack of acute articular rheumatism. He had a sore throat and a pain in his head which would shoot down to his left shoulder and to his finger tips, and also shot through his legs. The pain was particularly agonizing in the right leg whenever his knee joint was moved. This pain persisted for a month after being in the hospital. He said his leg was like a log from the time of his collapse on the straw. This was a hysterical symptom of some duration, for when the pains left him after a month in the hospital his right leg was paralyzed, with an anaesthesia of the skin of the whole leg. He was got up out of bed but he had a gait typical of hysterical monoplegia, and had to walk with a crutch. The use of this led to a crutch palsy, and after a month or so he had paralysis of the right arm, purely hysterical, and also accompanied with a superficial anaesthesia. These symptoms persisted for eight months before I examined him, at which time the power of both arm and leg was steadily improving with methods of re-education.

The mechanism for this conversion hysteria seems fairly plain. The patient was tired of the situation in which he found himself and was anxious to receive some sort of an injury which would incapacitate him for active service.  Then he had what was apparently an attack of acute arthritis in the right knee which caused him great pain whenever his leg moved.  The paralysis, which then developed, can be easily explained as a protective reaction, since it immobilized the knee joint.  The explanation for its persistence and for the development of the paralysis of the arm is equally simple.  These disabilities provided ample occasion for his continued absence from the front.  It may be added that these paralyses were accompanied by the typical, hysterical, mental attitude, for the patient was unable to imagine himself using his leg at all.

But this patient also showed other symptoms.  It has been mentioned that he wished for death and that he had had some nightmares of fighting.  He therefore was in the mental state prior to his rheumatism of a man who develops an anxiety condition, and had also begun to show some symptoms of it.  When he was removed to the hospital he began to have more severe nightmares, although he never had any anxiety symptoms during the day that were at all severe or noticeable.  Complicating the conversion hysteria, therefore, he had a mild anxiety state. This was always in the background, for the dreams became infrequent and less severe long before there was any improvement at all in his paralysis.

The following three cases represent the development of hysterical phenomena as a continuance of disabilities that are more or less organic.

CASE XX.  The patient is a private in the heavy artillery who enlisted in December, 1914, but did not reach France until March, 1916.  His history showed that he had some mild neurotic tendencies inasmuch as he was afraid of high places, uncomfortable in thunder-storms, and did not like to go into tunnels. In other respects he was quite normal and seemed to have an open personality· and to be quite sociable. He was happily married.

He enjoyed his work at the front tremendously and the severe strain of long continued duration produced no symptoms, not even subjective fatigue. On August 2, 1916, when he had been fighting for four months, he was buried by the earth thrown up from the explosion of a heavy shell, and suffered severe concussion. Consciousness, that he could remember, returned only after three weeks, and following that for about ten days he suffered from lapses of consciousness whenever he exerted himself in the slightest degree. For months he continued to be extremely weak. Soon after recovering consciousness for the first time he found that he was easily startled by sudden noises, but had only occasional nightmares of fighting, and absolutely no continuous anxiety during the day. He was, as is often the case after severe concussion, subject to almost constant tremors that were independent of any conscious anxiety. This "shakiness," as he termed it, continued whenever he made any exertion for some months, and he found that the only way that he could control it was to cross his legs and hold them stiffly in this position. At first, of course, he was too weak to stand. Later, when his strength had returned, he found that whenever he would attempt to get out of bed his legs would go immediately into an adductor spasm and shake violently. He was treated with no improvement whatever in general hospitals for some eleven months, and was then transferred to a special hospital where I saw him only for four days after he had been admitted there. The treatment given was to stretch forcibly the adductors of the thighs by pulling his feet apart. This was continued until the adductor muscles were exhausted and incapable of further contraction. He was then put on his feet and, being supported, was encouraged to walk. For the first time he was able to get one leg past the other. During the four days that had elapsed he had lost the spasm in his left thigh almost completely and was able with an effort to control that in his right. The tremors too had almost entirely disappeared. He felt himself that he would be quite well in a few days. This case is a dramatic example of how simple a matter it is to cure these hysterical symptoms, in spite of long duration, when once rational treatment is employed.

In connexion with this gait disturbance, it might be well to recall Case IX. This patient it will be remembered developed a similar condition of spasticity when he attempted to walk on leaving his bed for the first time. With him, too, the spasm developed as an effort to control the violent tremors of his legs, but these tremors were probably much more functional in origin than those present in the patient whose history has just been quoted.

CASE XXI. The patient is a private, aged 25, whose only neurotic tendencies had been a fear of lightning and of snow. He had, however, rather a poor personality, enjoying distinctly low ideals and being rather given to lying, although not at all in a malicious way. He enlisted in the regular army in 1911, but deserted before long and became a professional football player. When the war broke out he re-enlisted and went to France in September, 1914.

He fought for six months and claimed to have enjoyed this first period of fighting. It was terminated, however, by an accident when he fell into a deep dugout, fracturing both his ankles, and suffering frost-bite before he could be taken back to the hospital. This experience seems to have given him a distaste for the war. He was back in England for three or four months, and then did not wish to return to France so soon. Even on the way back he began to be frightened at the prospect. He was kept for two months in barracks and then went up the line. He approached the trenches feeling quite anxious and, on arrival, got immediately into a panic but was saved from further difficulties by being wounded through the thigh almost at once. This was a minor injury but it necessitated his remaining in a hospital for a couple of weeks. This hospital was exposed to occasional shell fire and the patient found that he was constantly starting at the noises and now and again had nightmares of fighting, although he would sleep through many nights without any disturbance whatever. He was then sent back to his base for some time, where he had no more nightmares at all, but was still "jumpy" when any particularly loud noise would occur. A fear of going back to the line had by this time become a settled part of his character. He was returned for three weeks to the trenches during which time he was constantly in fear but developed no symptoms whatever. This brief period of fighting was again terminated when he received some superficial wounds from fragments of a shell, and this time he was fortunate enough to be sent back to England for five months. He returned again in May, 1916, and fought till September. During this time one gathers that he tried hard to work up the symptoms of appendicitis and trench fever but was never able to convince the medical officer that there was anything serious the matter with him. He was frightened, of course, but always slept well and had no nightmares. In the middle of September he saw one of his comrades run over and crushed by a tank and, for the first time, he felt horror. From then on any sight of blood affected him. Two or three hours after this unpleasant experience he was shot in the right forearm (another flesh wound) which caused his removal to a dressing station and then to a rest camp. He was in the latter for two weeks, during which time he felt constantly afraid of returning to the trenches and was very loth to get better. From the rest camp he was sent to the base to join another battalion and was then thrown into the line again. He was there for three days, during which time he suffered considerably from his horror of bloodshed and from his constant fear. He was therefore much relieved when after only three days' fighting he fractured his left collar-bone and left wrist. He was sent back to a casualty clearing station, and was only too glad to give a pint and a half of his blood for transfusion as he was rewarded for this by being shipped home to England. After a few weeks his left arm came out of the splint, when he discovered (probably not without satisfaction) that his arm was paralyzed. He remained without the use of this limb for five months during which time all kinds of treatment were attempted. He was then sent to a special hospital where simple methods of re-education resulted quite quickly in the steady return of strength to his arm.

It is interesting to note that once his hysterical paralysis began to improve he developed some nightmares. This, presumably, indicates the strong resistance he felt to the idea of returning to the front.

The following case could perhaps be described as an atypical anxiety state but is probably better grouped with the hysterias inasmuch as tremors and weakness and digestive disturbances were more prominent than the signs of pure anxiety. The case is also important as it shows how poor a soldier the individual makes who up to the time of enlistment has been a highly neurotic individual. It is not improbable that his symptoms were atypical because he was suffering as much from a peace as from a war neurosis.

CASE XXII is a private, aged 23. He had always been nervous. As a child he would scream if left alone either day or night. He had such fear of falling that he could not approach a window. It required the greatest effort for him to enter a subway. He was afraid of lightning. He hated to see anybody fighting, and accidents made him sick. He would pant with anxiety if he heard fire-engine bells. He also had suffered from occasional bilious attacks. Frequently he dreamed that the house was on fire. When the Zeppelin raids began over London he was terrified by them. He was so seclusive that he had never made any friends with either sex, and had such poor stuff in him that his brothers called him a girl and not a boy.

This individual, so poorly adapted to civilian life, enlisted in October, 1915, and went to France four months later. The training in an artillery company did him good physically, but it led to further difficulties mentally and nervously. He could not make any friends and was constantly afraid of doing things wrong. Fear of the fighting, that was to come, increased steadily as the time grew near when he would have to go to the front. On reaching France he was at first back of the front line of trenches, and consequently he saw very little fighting for some time. Some of the enemy aeroplanes appeared, however, which scared him horribly, and for some nights he could not get to sleep thinking of them. For the first month he was busy carrying

rations and munitions from the rear up to the communication
trenches; then he began to work with his battery. For the first
three weeks the battery remained immune from attack; then
it was shelled. The patient was frightened and could not help
crying out "What a terrible one that was!" whenever a shell
came. He was promptly told to keep quiet but was unable to do
so. In subsequent bombardments he would listen attentively to
the successive reports from the guns, and convince himself that
the enemy. guns were coming closer. The first sight of the
wounded affected him so extremely that he almost cried,
although somehow or other he managed to get used to this
sufficiently for him to continue at work. From the time when
he first approached the line, however, he began to dream of the
enemy coming after him with bayonets. These nightmares of
course disturbed his sleep, and he also had great difficulty in
getting to sleep at all when he lay down to rest. Although he
got gradually worse he somehow or other managed to continue
in his ineffective way for some nine months. His battery was
finally relieved and sent to a rest camp where he at once felt a
little better. Then a false report came that the battalion was to
return to the front. The patient at once collapsed. He could
not stand, was shaking all the time, crying and vomiting. The
nightmares became so severe that he could not sleep at all for
four nights after his admission to a hospital. For some days also
he was able to keep nothing whatever on his stomach, and during
the six months that had elapsed since that time when I saw him
he had not eaten a single full meal. He was sent back to England
and treated in various hospitals. He improved twice, being able
once to walk from one bed to another, although he often fell with
giddiness, after which he would shake terribly and sweat pro-
fusely. This improvement lasted for a week. There was then
some talk of his being sent to a convalescent hospital. The
patient began to fear that, if he recovered, he would be sent back
to France, and although this was more a passing idea than a constant worry, it may explain the fact that he fell down again when
this transfer was imminent and was not able to get up again. He
was sent to the convalescent home, however, where he improved

again, this time with electrical treatment. He got so that he could walk but then pains developed in his back and across his hips which soon put a stop to his walking. He had been told that he would not be sent from the convalescent home to a special hospital unless he became worse again, and probably this is what caused the development of the pains. When I saw him he had been in this special hospital for ten days during which time he had become much less shaky although he was still unable to walk. He had a rigidity of the muscles along his spine and some diminishing signs of hyperthyroidism. His dreams had become much better—that is his nightmares of being bayoneted were tending to disappear, but he was troubled with other nightmares of the peace type; for instance he would dream that the hospital was on fire, or that Zeppelins were going to come. Once while sleeping on a balcony he dreamed that it collapsed but that he hung on to the edge with his fingers. He awoke screaming to the nurse to come and rescue him.

The following case shows how an anxiety state in an officer can be inhibited from further development when other symptoms develop—in this case symptoms of a gastric neurosis.

CASE XXIII. The patient is a lieutenant, aged 24. He had never had any illness in his life, but had always been of a high-strung nervous temperament. He was afraid of the dark as a child and had night terrors. These were mainly of falling into a huge funnel and being jammed in the bottom. He had had no fear of thunder-storms or of tunnels, but would become rather excited and could not trust himself if he were in a high place. He was shy with girls and saw nothing of them until he left school at 18, but thought that he had improved somewhat in this respect as he grew older—in fact he has recently become engaged. His social relationships with those of his own sex were apparently quite normal. It is important to note that he had always been sensitive to pain and more than normally sympathetic. Once when he was a boy a companion took him into a butcher's yard to see a pig killed. This upset him greatly and he felt excited for some time after.

He enlisted as a private in September, 1914, and reacted well to his training except that he was troubled with a little fear of being a coward in France. He conquered this, however, to the point of being able to look forward to the trial, and when he went there in March, 1915, he was pleased to find that his nerve was as good as that of the rest. He got used to being shelled quite quickly but found in the nine months of fighting, during which he served, that, so long as he was in perfect physical condition, he had the feeling that nothing could hurt him, but that whenever he became tired this conviction would disappear. After seven months of fighting he was exposed to a monotonous bombardment with howitzers for three days. He and his comrades were in an advanced "bay" and it was only a question of time before every man would be killed in all probability. Nothing happened to him, however, before he was relieved. He was calm mentally but could not stop shaking for three hours after leaving the trenches. Following this experience he was "jumpy" and felt disappointed in himself. He did not lose sleep, however, or have any nightmares, but found it gradually more difficult to control himself whenever a methodical bombardment was in progress. In December, 1915, he was sent back to England to receive training as an officer, which lasted for six months. He was glad of the rest but disappointed to find that it did not do him so much good as he had hoped. He went to work to have as good a time as possible because he expected that he would be killed when he went back to France. He was much more worried at the thought of going to pieces nervously than by any fear of death itself. He went back as lieutenant in June, 1916, and found that it cost more effort than before to control his fear. The strain of constantly encouraging his men told on him. He did not actually lose sleep, but always felt heavy when he awoke in the morning. Trench mortars were very active in his section of the line and the frightful explosions from them constantly upset him. His whole spirit grew weary of the war. So far his history is quite typical of the prodromal period of an anxiety state.

The sight of blood had not bothered him at any time, although seeing a man blown to bits or losing a comrade always upset him.

He felt distinctly encouraged when he saw dead Germans.  After being nearly four months in France as an officer a shell blew up a group of men right beside him.  One of them remained sitting down with his back against the wall of a trench and the patient thought that he was alive.  He went up to him and touched him on the helmet.  Immediately the whole back of the man's head rolled off and exposed the back of his eyes and his nose and teeth.  This sight gave the patient a terrible "turn."  He went into the dugout and trembled for several hours.  He did not feel any nausea but when the time next came to eat he discovered that he had absolutely no appetite, and from that time on it required a great effort to put any food in his mouth.  In describing this incident the patient emphasized the fact that he was merely a calm observer of the tragedy.  He felt that if the shell had knocked him over it would have given him some degree of relief.  From then on he began to feel horror of all bloodshed and was quite incapable of developing any excitement no matter how active the fighting might be.  He felt that all individuality in the struggle was lost and that it was a pure matter of siege warfare. He could gain no satisfaction in killing one or many of the enemy.  His sleep, however, was not interfered with and he had no nightmares.

While in this condition (October, 1916) he was transferred to Salonika.  There was no active fighting there, but sufficient exertion was demanded to cause fatigue, particularly since he was eating little or nothing.  In making a landing on the coast from the transport he got wet and had not an opportunity of changing his clothes for several days.  Shortly after this a neuralgic pain appeared in his mouth.  Previously, however, he had begun to suffer from flatulence.  The next symptom to develop was constipation, the faecal matter being foul, and he began to have nausea whenever his bowels did move.  Possibly as a result of the restricted diet, which was mainly canned beef and biscuits, pyorrhea began to develop.  Although he was thoroughly miserable his symptoms remained in the physical sphere, except once when an enemy airplane flew over the lines.  They fired at it with anti-aircraft guns, and this incident excited the patient so much that he knew his nerve was no better. After suffering for three weeks with neuralgia he asked to be sent to the hospital, which request was granted. He was there for three weeks, and then was sent to the base depot. The food was worse than any supplied previously and after three days he began to vomit and was sent to the hospital where he was put on a milk diet. As all tests were negative it 'was concluded that he was suffering from a gastric neurosis, and he was shipped to Malta where he was kept for three or four months and then sent home to England. While in Malta there was no improvement in his condition and he settled down to the belief that he was a confirmed invalid. In England he was put in a special hospital where he had improved slightly at the time that I saw him. His neuralgia had almost entirely left him and the vomiting had disappeared. He still had no appetite, however, and frequently suffered from nausea either before or after eating. Constipation was alternating with diarrhoea. Mentally he complained of a lack of interest and spontaneity. He said he had forgotten his education—that his youth and his eagerness were all gone. In explaining his poor adaptation to fighting he said that he thought that the strain told on him because of his imagination. It was impossible for him to keep the belief from his mind that every shell was meant for him.

In this case, therefore, we have a patient who had always had some neurotic tendencies although they had never incapacitated him during civilian life. One of these was an undue sensitiveness to cruelty or bloodshed. After some months of fighting the strain began to tell on him, his condition growing steadily worse, and it seems as if the normal development of his difficulties would have led to a typical anxiety state. Up to this time, however, he had always remained more or less immune to the horrors of war. Then suddenly a particularly fearful experience branded horror on his mind and symptoms of another kind developed at once. From then on the pathological tendencies seemed to flow in the direction of a gastric neurosis rather than in the ordinary channel of an anxiety state.

# CHAPTER IX

## HEART NEUROSES

In times of peace certain symptoms related to the function of the heart are frequent concomitants of anxiety conditions—in fact fear of death may be directly associated with fear that heart failure is imminent. Except for some rapidity of the pulse of which the patient is often not aware the typical war anxiety neurosis shows nothing of this tendency. There is, however, rather a large group of men who are invalided from the trenches with heart symptoms but who show no signs of valvular trouble. These cases have been termed "soldier's heart" or "disordered action of the heart." The cardinal symptoms of this cardiac trouble are weakness, shortness of breath, palpitation and dizziness. Not infrequently there is an area of hyperalgesia over or near the heart. Owing to the obvious analogy between these symptoms and those presented by the cardiac difficulties of civilians suffering from anxiety it has been suggested that the "disordered action of the heart" is really a form of the war anxiety neurosis. Some internists who have been engaged in treating these cases make the statement that 50 per cent. are really neurotics. The word neurotic is one, of course, that is used in widely varying senses. By some it is an adjective to describe any physical symptom that has not an obvious physical cause, being therefore equivalent to functional disturbance. The narrower sense of the term implies a mental condition which shows itself in certain types of reaction and produces or tends to produce, somehow or other, physical symptoms. Those who use the term in the narrower sense find, for instance, that prior to the appearance of active symptoms the patient gives a history of being subjected to some mental conflict or having suffered from some mental shock. Neurologists or psychiatrists who have this view would not call disturbances of the ductless glands, e.g., hyperthyroidism, neuroses.

Work which has been done by Frazer and Wilson at the Hampstead Hospital (for heart cases) in London seems to indicate that a large number of these cases are suffering from some irregularity of function in the endocrinic or vegetative nervous systems. The administration of very small quantities of adrenalin, for instance, they find to produce excessive excitement, great pallor, discomfort and real collapse, although there is no change in the pulse rate. On the other hand, small doses of apocodein result in flushing even to the point of erythema accompanied by extreme tachycardia. Atropin on the other hand even in full doses produces no effects whatever. A few patients, who were treated experimentally with small doses of pineal extracts, showed vomiting and collapse. These results would certainly seem to indicate that these patients were suffering from some definite disturbances of the mechanism which regulates the action of the heart and are therefore definitely organic, although not suffering from valvular diseases. This view is sustained by the histories which show as a rule that these individuals have never been capable of a normal amount of exertion—for instance, they have been unable to play any games that demanded endurance, although capable of taking part in such milder sports as golf. It has been found that this lack of vitality of the heart can be quickly determined by an "exercise test." The patient's pulse is counted and he is then made to go briskly up a flight of thirty steps. His pulse is taken immediately and then again after he has rested for two minutes. The normal individual will show a rise of 40 or perhaps 45 in the pulse rate after this exertion, but this falls after two minutes' rest back to the original rate or to within 10 or at most 15 of it. Patients who suffer from "disordered action of the heart," however, may show an increase of rate of 60 or more and the pulse does not slow down again after two minutes' rest, or at least will slow only in slight measure.

In order to see whether from a psychiatric standpoint they

were really "neurotic" I examined some ten cases with a view to determining what their mental and emotional history had been. These cases were very kindly picked out for me by Dr Wilson as most likely to be purely neurotic. I was able to make diagnosis of a true neurosis in only two of these cases, and in all of them a prediction as to the result of the exercise test was found to be accurate when reference was made to the notes on the patient. Although this is of course too small a number to make any deductions in the form of percentages, the results are nevertheless sufficiently striking to justify one in assuming that the majority of the patients who suffer from "disordered action of the heart" are not neurotics in the narrow sense of the word. A few illustrative cases may be quoted. The first gives an example of the purely organic and non-neurotic type of disease.

CASE XXIV. The patient is a private, aged 29, who enlisted in February, 1917, in a labour battalion and did clerical work in a casualty clearing station in France. He had never been able to keep up any severe exertion and for this reason had to restrict his activities in athletics. All his life he was subject to palpitations of the heart and would frequently wake up with a choking feeling at night, although he had not had any bad dreams that he could recall. When his sleep was thus disturbed he would have a terrible sensation, with difficulty in getting himself fully awake. On the other hand he seems to have been emotionally a normal individual. He suffered from no night terrors as a child and had none of the ordinary neurotic fears or sensibilities except a slight giddiness in high places, which is a symptom that affects almost everyone whether he be otherwise neurotic or not. He was never given to worry. He had been a normal mischievous boy, had never had any shyness with either sex, and at the time when I examined him had been married for five years and professed himself happier since his marriage than he had ever been before.

In his work in the casualty clearing station he was of course exposed to shell fire at times. This bothered him only temporarily. The sight of the wounds also affected him with horror for a short time only, after which he became fully accustomed

8—2

to both forms of strain. He had no nightmares. On the other hand the physical exertion that was necessary told on him gradually more and more and his previous symptoms of palpitation and nocturnal choking got so bad that he could not continue working and he was sent to a hospital. All during this time he had no anxiety whatever and was bitterly disappointed to find that he had to stop "doing his bit." The exercise test showed that he had an initial pulse of 120 which rose to 168 after exertion and fell only to 144 after two minutes' rest.

The following two cases exhibited the more neurotic reaction.

CASE XXV. The patient is a private, aged 20. As a child he had night terrors and was subject to sleep walking until 8 years of age. He was always anxious during thunder-storms and giddy in high places, although he admitted no uncomfortableness in tunnels. He made some boy friends but was very shy with girls and not at all mischievous. He had never had any serious disease although he had a slight attack of tonsilitis at the age of 6 from which he recovered without any subsequent complications. He was able to play games as a boy and was particularly fond of football, but gave it up when he was 14 because he found that he was getting short of breath. Considering that he was capable of exertion prior to this time, it is not impossible that this dyspnoea coming on at the time of puberty was a neurotic symptom, since so many neuroses begin at this time.

The training did him good as he made more friends than he ever had before. At first he found himself considerably fatigued with the efforts demanded of the recruits, but he improved in this as the training went on. When he reached the front he was frightened only temporarily by the shells but never could accustom himself to all the horrors of war. He fought for seven months, when he was invalided home for six months with "septic poisoning." On his return to the front in July, 1916, he felt nervous again at first but got used to it once more. In September, he began getting pains in his side, for which he was sent to the hospital. There he had no fever and the pains quickly disappeared and remained absent while he was convalescent for a month.  As soon as he returned to the trenches, however, they reappeared.  His condition grew severe enough to justify hospital treatment in December, 1916, at which time he was away from the trenches for three months.  On his return to them again he held out only three weeks, and for the next three months, at the end of which time I saw him, he had been travelling from hospitals to convalescent camps and back again.

Evidence of there being definitely neurotic prodromata is furnished by the following information which he gave.  Before any heart symptoms developed he had become "nervous."  He was "jumpy" during the day and frequently awoke at night with a start.  He also had difficulty in getting to sleep.  He was thoroughly dissatisfied with his situation and had reached the point where he hoped that he might receive some incapacitating wound.  This situation is therefore identical with that which one usually meets in the history of the typical conversion hysteria, and it is also like that rather than resembling the anxiety state in that he had no desire for death and no thoughts of suicide.  The symptoms began after he had been in this state of mind for some time, and consisted at first merely of a pain in the region of his heart.  The subsequent difficulties with palpitation, shortness of breath and weakness developed later on.  There is, therefore, nothing in this case that points definitely to any organic condition, and, on the other hand, the evidence does seem to indicate that the heart symptoms were essentially hysterical in nature.  This is confirmed by the exercise test which showed him to have a pulse of 75 before exertion, 108 immediately after running up the thirty steps, and only 84 when he had rested two minutes.

CASE XXVI.  The patient is a gunner, aged 35, an Australian. He seems to have had a distinctly neurotic make-up.  As a child he had night terrors with dreams of falling.  He was always horrified at the sight of blood and was afraid of thunder-storms, high places, tunnels and horses.  He does not seem to have been a normal mischievous boy, and when he grew older was shy with both sexes.  He had had only one love affair, which he broke off in 1911 for no apparent reason.  His training was of benefit physically but not mentally or nervously and he showed no increased sociability during it. His first service was in Egypt. On the way there he developed a fear of shipwreck which was not shared by his companions. He was in Egypt for some months, and although there was no fighting, he found the weather hot and uncomfortable and he suffered from occasional palpitations and "sinking feelings" which he ascribed to the heat.

He was transferred to the French front in May, 1916. In his initial experience of being shelled he became first terrified and then dull and depressed. He was horrified by the sight of blood and would think about it whenever he was not busy. He never was able to reach the point of enjoying any of the fighting. He soon began having peculiar sensations when going off to sleep as if he were sinking, or that his soul was leaving his body, and he would have to sit up in bed two or three times to get rid of this queer feeling. He also would awaken with sudden starts, although not having any memory of a bad dream. Things got gradually worse and then he began to have nightmares of "things" (mainly shells) falling on him. He would try to get away from them, but could not. His sleep consequently began to be much worse, and he worried for fear he would not be able to stick it out. He wished that death might come, but never had a hope of receiving an incapacitating wound. He frequently thought of suicide. At the beginning of May, 1917, he was blown off his feet by a shell. This did not injure him physically apparently but disturbed him mentally a great deal. From that time on he felt that the shells were being aimed at him, and four days after this experience he developed a pain in his side, trembling and difficulty in breathing. He said his throat swelled up and he felt as if he were going to choke. He attributed this to being gassed, although he had not been exposed to this any more than had his companions, who showed no symptoms of it. As he had been wishing for death it is not unnatural that he should have looked on this choking sensation as a forerunner of death and he quickly concentrated most of his fear on this symptom which naturally made it much worse. He claims that it once was so bad that he "went black in the face" and he got so short of breath and tremulous that the bombardier sent him back to a hospital. Once in the hospital he grew weaker and weaker and was so terrified by his dreams that he would scream aloud on awakening from them. After six weeks in a special heart hospital all the symptoms directly related to the heart cleared up although he was still troubled occasionally with suffocating feelings during the night which continued to frighten him, the fear being always of instant dissolution. Nightmares with a war content had entirely disappeared, although he still had occasional dreams of falling. There was no evidence of any organic trouble which could have caused the feeling of suffocation. The exercise test showed an initial pulse of 96 running up to 168 after exercise but falling to 84 after two minutes' rest.

The history of the following patient is interesting as it seems to demonstrate the existence of both organic and neurotic factors. It appears that he had the prodromal symptoms of a neurosis the further development of which was essentially organic. As has been said before, a large part of the motivation of any neurosis comes from a desire to be rid of trench life. When any real occasion for absence from the firing line appears there is therefore little reason left for the development or continuance of the true neurosis.

CASE XXVII. The patient is a private, aged 19, who enlisted in the territorials in January, 1914, but did not reach France until September, 1916. As a child he had had night terrors and some fear of the dark which persisted up to the time when he enlisted at the age of 16. He had no fear of thunder-storms but was giddy in high places and would break out into a cold sweat and tremble whenever he had to go through a tunnel. He suffered from enuresis until 10 years of age and from puberty onward had considerable worry about emissions. He does not seem to have been particularly seclusive so far as his social adaptations are concerned. He was good at games but always had a tendency to shortness of wind. When he began training he was, of course, only 16 years of age and had considerable difficulty in carrying his pack at first. Then he got used to it and felt distinctly stronger. When he reached France he found the life in the trenches distasteful. He could not accustom himself to the horrors around him and worried over them constantly. He was never able to make himself perfectly indifferent to bombardment. He began quite soon to wish that he might be killed or, at any rate, be removed from the trenches for some cause or other. He had no nightmares, however, and did not lose any sleep. Then pains developed under his heart, accompanied by shortness of breath, palpitation, dizziness, and a feeling of faintness. He connected these heart symptoms with the previous "weakness of his bladder" from which he had suffered (enuresis) but did not worry about them more than he did about the shells[1].

The medical officer sent him off duty several times for treatment of his heart trouble. After three months in the trenches and having been sent to the hospital for short periods several times he developed "trench feet" and was sent back to England. His heart condition then attracted attention and he was transferred to a special hospital where I saw him. On admission the pulse test was positive—that is, the rate did not diminish as it normally does after two minutes' rest. After being treated for several months with graduated exercises he was capable of going through the heaviest routine and the pulse test had become negative. It is therefore likely that the cardiac mechanism had recovered very largely in a purely organic sense. The patient still insisted, however, that his heart trouble was not getting any better. One might therefore be justified in suspecting that this patient was rather consciously hoping for a persistence of his symptoms.

Although the heart cases examined for the purpose of this report were too few in number to justify any finality in the discussion of the mental mechanisms involved, it may be suggested that there are perhaps two types that correspond roughly to the

[1] Although not a final diagnostic point by any means, this emotional attitude of indifference toward the heart symptoms is suggestive of an organic rather than a functional condition. The ideas of heart disease and death are closely allied; so we find as a rule that a fear of death is frequently associated with neurotic heart symptoms—in fact, as in the last case, the neurotic "cause of death" is apt to occasion more fear than a real cause.

anxiety and the conversion hysteria groups. Some heart cases like Case **XXVI** seem to have a very strong colouring of anxiety, and this is associated with a desire for death as a form of relief before the actual appearance of the symptoms. In the other group as represented by Case **XXV** a wish for an incapacitating wound rather than for death is present in a prodromal state and when the heart symptoms develop they are looked on more objectively as a disease and are not accompanied by the same anxiety. This feeble emotional reaction to the symptoms is therefore closely parallel to, if not identical with, the phenomena of the conversion hysteria. There are of course no statistics available as to the number of purely neurotic heart conditions that develop at the front. It is safe to say, however, that they form an insignificant group numerically when compared to the anxiety states and common conversion hysterias. The reason for this is probably to be found in the fact that there is nothing that is much more painful both mentally and physically than symptoms of heart trouble which are so commonly associated with idea of death. The neurotic, therefore, who is unconsciously on the search for some relief is much more apt to wish for death by a shell or a bayonet than for the more protracted and painful struggle that precedes death by heart failure.

# CHAPTER X

## GENERAL PSYCHOLOGICAL CONSIDERATIONS

It may be well to summarize what has been said earlier in this report by a few generalizations as to the psychological mechanisms at work in the production of the war neuroses. The most fundamental factor is of course the resistance of the officer or soldier to the warfare in which he is forced to engage. A striking feature of these conditions is that this resistance can be present in the patient's mind consciously and still operate unconsciously in the production of symptoms, which is a phenomenon rarely if ever met with in civilian practice. It is probably more accurate to say that the general antagonism to the situation remains conscious, while some specific wish for relief begins to operate unconsciously and reaches expression when a situation develops that facilitates its transformation into a symptom.

That these transformations should differ so widely in their nature as do simple hysterical symptoms and the mental torture of an anxiety state demands some brief discussion. The first clue to be followed in solving this mystery is the striking fact that the vast majority of those suffering from the pure anxiety state are officers, while the conversion hysterias are almost entirely confined to the privates and non-commissioned officers. The most obvious difference between these two groups of men lies in their intelligence, and here we find an analogy with the experience of civilian practice. The common conversion hysterias are met with in times of peace very largely among the lower and more poorly educated classes, while more intelligent people are apt to be free from them. One explanation of this may be that the modern educated man knows enough of neurology to realize, even if it be in a vague way, that paralysis comes from injury to a nerve or the central nervous system at some distance from the site of the paralysis. The intelligent layman, for example, knows that if he breaks his wrist the forearm and hand are apt to be painful and consequently there may be some weakness in the forearm and hand, but he does not expect that all the muscles involved in wrist movements will be paralyzed. He would expect this to occur more probably after a paralytic stroke, injury to the spinal cord or an accident to a nerve in the upper arm. The ignorant dispensary or hospital patient, on the other hand, has a definite association in his mind between local symptoms and local functions and he has little if any conception of nervous control from a distance. An example of this failure to localize function correctly is the popular use of the term "a strong wrist" when a strong forearm is really meant.

But the difference between officers and men does not begin and end with intelligence and education. That one is a leader and another a follower is equally the result of a difference in ideals and emotional attitude. The private's ambition is not to think for himself but to follow orders implicitly and to sink his own personality so far as that may be possible. If a dangerous project is on foot the private is not in a situation to decide whether he will join in with it or use some caution—he is merely faced with the alternatives of obeying orders or being court-martialled. The officer on the other hand has to a larger measure the responsibility of individual decision. He has to make up his mind whether he is or is not going to give a certain order—whether he will or will not expose himself to danger. Moreover, it is his duty not only to be courageous himself and to prevent the thoughts of his personal danger from disturbing his judgment, but he must also act before his men as to inspire them and give an example of indifference to all the hazards of war. This implies that the officer must be endowed with higher ideals than the private soldier. It is to this more than to any other factor probably that we may ascribe the difference between their clinical histories, when war neuroses develop. The officer who feels his responsibility in the great struggle which the war represents is prepared to do all he can for the country, even to the point of facing death itself, but before that final release may come his mind stops at no other excuse. When fatigue and the horrors of war grow on him, therefore, he does not let his fancy play with any failure to meet his full responsibilities but looks forward rather to making the supreme sacrifice, namely, that of dying for his country. The private, on the other hand, is willing to accept an order to leave the trenches with the same or even greater willingness than he will obey an order to advance against the enemy. The most obvious occasion for an order to go back of the line is, of course, a wound which will incapacitate him from further active service and it is therefore "a Blighty one" for which he yearns.

The transformation of these wishes into symptoms is the next point to be considered. The fate of the private is a simple matter. He wishes for some physical disability and when the appropriate physical or mental accident occurs some physical disability appears, that is to say, a conversion hysteria develops which is, so far as he can see, purely a physical disability, and his mental attitude toward the symptom is very much like that which any man exhibits toward a wound or some somatic disease. The determination of the particular symptom can usually be traced to some previous illness, when the function in question was organically disturbed. The conversion of the wish for death into the anxiety symptom is, however, not so obvious a matter. In general one may say that nightmares, which are the most distinctive feature of the anxiety state, do not seem to develop until the wish for death has appeared. It is possible, therefore, that the unconscious mind seizes on that in the environment which is most likely to occasion death and makes the patient dream of this danger. The "wish-fulfilment," therefore, in the dream of being shelled or bayoneted may be ascribed to the wish for death which may previously have been rather diffuse and now becomes specifically allied with one particular form of mortal danger. To account for the presence of anxiety in these dreams, when there has been previously a calm desire for death, is a more difficult matter. The only explanation seems to be that emotional reactions in dreams seem to represent the natural reactions of the individual, as an individual, rather than of the socialized being who is burdened with a feeling of moral responsibility. It is of course a commonplace that we constantly dream of performing acts which we would never indulge in when we are awake, out of consideration for the feelings of others, or out of respect for laws or conventions. In a somewhat similar way our emotional reaction in dreams is determined by our more selfish attitude toward the situation presented in the dream. It is of course a perfectly normal thing for any man to be afraid of a high explosive shell or of a bayonet; the instinct of self-preservation bids him be afraid. This too is his initial reaction when first exposed to such dangers, but he soon learns to inhibit this fear during the daytime because he knows that it is his duty to be indifferent to these dangers. This inhibition is lifted during sleep, however, and consequently his emotional reaction during the dream is that which any civilian would have when placed in such an extremity. Another factor may possibly also enter in. Fear, as has been said, is a protective reaction. Now the individual has to protect himself from real dangers not only from without but from the unconscious cravings which are at variance with his social standards. All the protective emotions of dreams are therefore probably operating in part to keep the unconscious tendencies in subjection—in other words, to keep them unconscious. It is for this reason that any man is often most fearful of that which he unconsciously most desires.

The unconscious wish for death by some definite agency operates in many cases at first during sleep but soon it begins to show itself in the daytime. Unconsciously desirous of being hit by a shell, the patient's attention is more attracted to bombardment than it previously was, consequently his thoughts become focused willy nilly upon it. It is then that the instinctive protective reaction of fear develops, perhaps in order to make the individual shun this danger. The patient loses the ability to gauge the direction of shells by their sounds, which gives a beautiful example of how the unconscious works at cross purposes from the conscious mind. The patient has consciously no fixed and constant desire to be hit by a shell. Unconsciously he has, however; so in the fatigued condition from which he suffers, the unconscious warps his judgment, making every shell the fulfilment of the unconscious wish.

The foregoing speculations as to the psychological stages in the formation of anxiety symptoms refer to those cases where nightmares precede diurnal fear. This does not always happen; in fact, it is probably of rarer occurrence than the reverse. There is no reason to suppose that there is any essential difference in mechanism between the two types of cases. The smaller group is chosen as a paradigm merely because unconscious motivation and individualistic reactions are always more easily observed in dreams than in the reactions of waking life.

It is now more or less of an axiom that unconscious factors retain their power very largely because of their remaining unconscious, and so beyond the sphere of influence of the individual's judgment. This is a factor of no small importance in the production of the anxiety states. The fear which the patient feels must be repressed. He is ashamed of showing any evidence of cowardice before either his men or his brother officers. He is therefore the subject of a conflict which he must fight alone. He knows that he has at least a tendency to be afraid, but he also knows that he can maintain the respect of his men and officer friends so long as he keeps that fear to himself. He is constantly repressing this most natural reaction and there is accumulated, naturally enough, a stronger and stronger tendency for active exhibitions of fear. It is this which probably accounts for two phenomena. The first is that when the patient is sent back from the trenches to the hospital and the occasion for this repression removed there is almost invariably a sudden increase in the severity of the symptoms. The second is that an opportunity for the frank discussion of a man's fear with his physician is often the occasion for his "getting a good deal off his chest" and leads to marked improvement in his condition.

A few remarks on the psychological role of concussion may not be out of place. In many patients in whom there have been gradually accumulating difficulties not sufficient to incapacitate the patient there is a sudden increase of symptoms following even a mild concussion. This is of course quite obviously the result of organic injury to the brain, but how this affects mental mechanisms should be considered. As has just been said, the unconscious seems to be a prominent factor in the actual production of symptoms. Normally, the unconscious is kept under such severe repression that no ideas are allowed to come into consciousness which are not fully adapted to the situation at hand, so that the reactions of the individual are in keeping with his natural standards of behaviour. This repression, however, is closely related to the higher mental functions, and for its perfect operation demands the fullest degree of both intellectual and moral judgment. Any injury to the brain naturally affects its more specialized functions first and more severely than it does those functions which we term "habitual" or instinctive. Hence, in the low state of mental tension consequent on cerebral injury the higher functions are in abeyance and the unconscious and instinctive tendencies can readily gain the upper hand. The situation with concussion is therefore—only in a psychological sense, of course—analogous to that of a mental shock. A purely psychic trauma so confuses the patient's ordinary mental processes that his critical judgment is for the time being impaired, and the unconscious has an opportunity for fuller expression than it previously enjoyed. Both concussion and mental shocks are by their nature sudden. We see also many cases in which there is a gradual increase in the severity of symptoms. It is not at all impossible that modern warfare produces conditions of such extreme neuropsychic fatigue that mental tension may be lowered thereby to that same level of inefficiency that occurs acutely with concussion or psychic trauma. This process is necessarily more gradual with the unconscious developing symptoms in inverse proportion to the weakening strength of the critical factors.

Throughout this report there has been considerable stress laid on the psychological aspects of the war neuroses. Inasmuch as it seems certain that purely physical factors play a larger role than they commonly do in times of peace in the production of functional nervous disturbances, this constant emphasis of the mental aspects of the neuroses demands some apology. The reason for it is a purely practical one. The treatment of these conditions, in so far as it demands the attention of specialists, must be almost purely psychological, or, to put the matter in a somewhat more accurate form, it may be said, perhaps, that every method of treatment instituted must be carefully considered in the light of its probably psychological effect. The physical factors, although of the utmost importance, are beyond our present capacity to change specifically. The best we can do, failing knowledge as to what they really are, is to meet them symptomatically with such simple measures as rest, diet, catharsis or sedation. It is only the physician who constantly maintains the psychological standpoint, however, who will be consistently successful in treating the war neuroses.

# CHAPTER XI

## PROPHYLAXIS

In conclusion it may be well to speak briefly of means that may be taken to prevent in future such terrible strains being made on the efficiency of fighting forces as the neuroses have produced in all the armies at present at war. The first method which naturally comes to mind is the removal at the time of enlistment of all men who are not adapted to fighting. This is, of course, a simple recommendation but one that demands keen judgment and wide outlook on the part of those who would put it into operation. One difficulty is inseparable from the problems of war itself. It must be obvious to every reader that the vast majority of cases quoted in this report show men who are well adapted to civil life but capable only to a limited degree of enduring the strain of modern warfare. The sad fact is also plain that the very qualities which may be the greatest assets to the civilian, and to the country in which he lives, may be just those characteristics which are most apt to jeopardize complete adaptation to trench warfare. I need only mention independence of judgment and a strong feeling of sympathy for those in pain, to make it clear that the ideal soldier must be more or less of a natural butcher, a man who can easily submit to the domination of intellectual inferiors. Whether men who are more valuable to the State as civilians than they are as soldiers, should be drafted into an army or not, is, fortunately, not a question for a physician examining recruits to decide. It is his duty, rather, to make up his mind, after an examination of any given applicant, whether the chances of that man's competency in the firing line will be sufficiently good to justify the money which the government will spend in feeding, clothing and training him.

It goes without saying that all men should be eliminated who
show marked psychopathic tendencies or who are obviously
psychoneurotic at the time of examination. On the other hand,
I have been much impressed with the large number of cases
(many of which are not reported here) that I have had an opportunity of examining who gave a history of previous breakdowns
or of having had tendencies toward psychoneurotic reactions in
their past life, but who nevertheless adapted themselves well to
training and fought well for many months, some of them indefinitely. I am therefore forced to the belief that there is in
military discipline a powerful therapeutic agency and that not
only the country as a whole, but many individuals, would lose
a great deal if they were denied service in the army simply
because they could show a history of some psychoneurotic disturbances in the past.

The problem, then, would reduce itself to a matter of gauging
the probable persistence and severity of such tendencies, which
is a difficult matter. No one of course who is ill-adapted to
civilian life at the time of enlistment should be considered.
Those patients who have given a history of such tendencies as
night terrors, fear of the dark, fear of the underground or fear
of thunder-storms, and who present no evidence of having out-
grown these tendencies, who are still in considerable measure incapacitated by them—all such persons are probably poor risks
from the army standpoint. Again it is practically certain that
any individual who is in times of peace temporarily incapacitated
by sights of cruelty, bloodshed, accidents, etc., is very unlikely
to have any but the briefest resistance to the constant strain
imposed by the inevitable horrors of war. Such symptoms as
giddiness in high places are so universal as to have practically
no significance when occurring alone. If it were practicable
much more finality in the physician's judgment could be given
if he had an opportunity of examining recruits twice. In his
first examination he could pick out doubtful cases and then re-
examine them after some months of training in order to discover
whether the military life had had a salutary or a deteriorating
effect on them. If they had improved they would probably be

good risks. If they had not improved, however, it would be highly improbable that their experience at the front would be anything but temporary. Although I have seen many cases showing neurotic tendencies who improved under training and became excellent soldiers, I have not seen one who failed to improve under training whose condition became better when he was actually in the firing line.

The next problem in connexion with prophylaxis has to do with lightening so far as possible the strain that is inevitable in trench warfare. It is of course an easy matter for the physician to say that the soldier must have frequent relief from duty and be given all possible distractions, and equally easy for the staff officers to reply that such coddling of the men is incompatible with the conduct of a campaign. Obviously this problem is at once both a military and a medical one. At the present time the line officers of the British Army are as acutely aware of the necessity for rest and distraction as are the physicians, and the reason for this is that they have discovered that no matter how much men may be forced and no matter how willing they may be to continue in the trenches they nevertheless become inefficient when subjected to more than a certain amount of fatigue. If at all feasible, a system of relief should be worked out in conference between psychiatrists and the staff. If also practicable, a certain laxity in the arrangements should be left whereby psychiatrists might be allowed the privilege of removing certain men from the trenches earlier than they would their fellows. If possible, this would be of great military advantage, as the history of many patients shows that when they have an opportunity to rest they quickly recover from the premonitory symptoms of a war neurosis and return to fight again quite competently. Once the disease has progressed beyond a certain point, however, there seems to be no return except after a long period of treatment. The best criterion I have been able to discover for permanence of symptoms is the presence of repeated nightmares of actual fighting. I was not able to find a single patient who had once shown these symptoms and subsequently improved without regular and protracted treatment. These remarks refer of course more particularly to the anxiety states than to the conversion hysterias. If all the private soldiers who complain of the milder degree of resistance to the trenches, which so many of these men show before the actual hysteria begins—if all these men were allowed to go back into rest camps there would probably be very little army left. On the other hand, the officers who break down with anxiety conditions, if they are good officers and of value to the army, are men who would be loth to leave their duty unless ordered to do so. It goes without saying that all forms of comfort and distraction, particularly the presence of palatable food and drink, are of importance from a medical standpoint in the present war as they never have been before. Where every factor seems to operate in making it hard for the soldier to maintain his adaptation—his pleasure in the service—it is essential that his difficulties should be reduced to a minimum, and that, on the other hand, he should be furnished with every possible means for giving him that pleasure which would distract his mind from all that is unpleasant and horrible around him.

Finally, when men are sent back to rest camps in order to recover from their fatigue it would be highly desirable that they should receive an examination before they return to active duty again. As has been shown in a number of cases in this report, the prospect of returning to duty, when recovery has not been complete, is frequently the occasion for utter discouragement and consequent collapse. In a war that may last for years an extra week or even an extra month of absence from the trenches is less loss to the army than is that which is occasioned by the protracted convalescence which follows only a week, perhaps, of efficient service. Here again then the problem is reduced to a question of adapting individual treatment to the military necessities which consider all men alike.